THE POLITICAL GUT

RESET YOUR REALITY

BRETT CASPER

PURE LUCK LIBRAY
NEW YORK | BANGKOK | OJAI

QUANTUM NUTRIENTS,
TWO BRAINS, UPSIDE-DOWN DIETS

Dedicated to
my mother
(1950 - 2023)

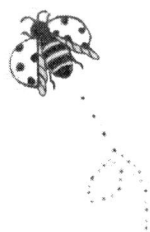

CONTENTS

PREFACE

One day in early Spring 2010 I opened my first bottle of kombucha, GT's Synergy. It was new in NYC at the time. I'd heard that kombucha was good for hangovers and I was really hungover. I remember the day exactly. It was a grey, cloudy day and the bottle had a big round, bright orange $5 sticker on the cap.

One Korean deli in Soho was selling it at the time. And so I kinda just chugged all 16oz. To my surprise, I felt a lot better, almost right away. Most notably my headache went away and my energy improved. This one solitary decision, seemingly innocuous at the time, changed the course of my life forever. It also reset my reality.

At the time I had been working as a professional artist with celebrities and luxury brands. As you could guess, there is a lot of partying involved with this lifestyle. So I started regularly picking up my $5 kombucha at the Korean deli to cure my hangovers.

That summer I had a British roommate sublet my spare bedroom. One day she brought home a kombucha kit and made kombucha. I had the same realization everyone else has. It's cheaper to brew my own! I already had a massive collection of tea since I'm fascinated by it.

And so I made 3 gallons of peach peony in an old, brown, glass milk jug. Which I found at the Junk store in Williamsburg. Surprisingly, it was delicious and had a freshness to it, like pop rocks in my mouth, sparkly and delightful to drink. The best part was that I could make any flavor I wanted.

After that, I started drinking kombucha regularly. Suddenly I began feeling like I would be healthier if I ate less meat. We love to BBQ, so steaks, burgers, and hot dogs were on the menu often. Not to mention the reubens, Italian subs, kebabs, and so many meaty choices in NYC. I made the decision and stopped eating meat for a year. It was a good experience and I learned a lot about how meat was affecting my personality. There's a chemical fed to slaughterhouse animals called Ractopamine.

I then started thinking a lot about how what we consume in turn controls our world view and personality. If just one bottle of fermented tea filled with bacteria could affect my personality and mood. How are all of the other chemicals and messaging really affecting my life through my decision making processes, mood and energy levels.

Over a decade later, research shows more and more, the bacterias in our gut control us. Our thoughts, decisions, mood, clarity, energy levels, fear response and even the voices in our head. I had the same question I think everyone grapples with daily. Do I choose to ignore this fact of life?

Or should I set out to understand how it controls me? I imagine that most people are like me and don't like being manipulated behind their backs. After drinking this first bottle of kombucha it was like a light switch was turned on. In an effort to discover my true self, I began my search for what I call true objectivity.

True objectivity to me was being able to guide my decision making processes by minimizing any outside influences from inputs like food, drugs, advertising and media. Essentially, testing our notion of free will. I want to be making decisions as close to gut level instinct as possible. What happened was that I ended up eliminating all the voices in my head. Thus, discovering an entirely new reality. One I controlled completely.

In the end I cut out all sugar, alcohol, drugs, meat, processed foods, chemicals and preservatives. To the point where I am eating an entirely organic diet that consists solely of spring water, fruits, vegetables, grains, eggs, greens, nuts, olive oil and occasional portions of fish. I even cut out caffeine and stopped drinking kombucha. Going full circle.

I never felt better in my life. Never have I had more energy and really felt high on life. Just by changing my diet. My personality changed completely and so did my outlook. The final ingredient was meditation.

Because you have to control your mind, for your mind and body to work as one. This is really important.

My aim with this book is to show you what I've learned. More importantly, how you can do it yourself. Everyone should be able to experience the freedom I feel. So I'm going to turn the pyramid upside-down and break it down bit by bit. Starting off slowly and working my way through each level, building.

I go into details, citing scientific research and providing personal anecdotes. Pointing out exactly how the current food and political systems are intertwined to keep us from making decisions in our best interests. How this is all tied to your gut health. How we are being programmed daily with food and messaging. Detailing how it is affecting our energy, and most importantly how to protect yourself and reset your reality. Each chapter gets denser and more provocative than the last. I am going to challenge what you believe to be reality.

Throughout the book I share the myriad of things that I have learned about the American food system and how it correlates from politics and capitalism directly to your health. Helping you to have a clearer view, to make better everyday choices. I read the research papers and did the homework for you.

Not only that. I spent 2 years during COVID lockdowns doing research working as an Instacart Shopper. While everyone was sitting home. I was spending 7 days a week in all types of supermarkets. I got to know every product and its ingredients very well. The one thing that stood out most.

If you buy something processed into a package in the United States it's nearly impossible to avoid corn syrup, sugar or one of the other 56 legalized versions of sweeteners. Cutting out sugar 100% from my diet was one of the most difficult tasks to fulfill. Now, if I consume anything with sugar in it. I can feel the effects of the sugar right away. I can't focus and feel antsy. Scientists say they still can't figure out what is causing the rise in ADHD.

Living in 4 countries, and traveling to 28 and counting, has really helped give me objectivity and put things in perspective for me. Experiencing new cultures has given me room for comparison. When seeing many versions of something. You can put them side by side and do what the human brain does best. Look for inconsistencies. Enabling critical thought. Because well, you don't know what you don't know.

As the former United States Secretary of Defense Donald Rumsfeld famously said, there are "known unknowns" and "unknown unknowns." If you've never known how it is to feel when eating healthy, you only know what you know. Not only that, you only know who you are as *that* person. We are born into paradigms. And have no comparison and therefore by extension, lack objectivity.

You may be shocked to find out. What you believe to be reality now, may not be the same reality when you finish reading this book. We owe it to our children and future generations to be custodians of possibility and good health.

Henry Kissenger, former United States secretary of state and national security advisor said, "Control food and you control people." And that's my reason for writing this book. I want to communicate important knowledge that at first seems unrelated, but when you put it all together a very clear picture emerges. This information is sometimes buried on purpose at most, and hard to find at least. And then there's the information made with intent to obfuscate. For many, the hardest part is making sense of it all.

What I've done is connect the seemingly disparate elements illustrating the larger picture. This book will give you more power and knowledge over your future, diet and health than you have ever had before. That is my promise to you.

I sincerely believe each person has the power to change the world. First by making the change they want to see within themselves.

CHAPTER ONE

Tea

A very long time ago in my early twenties I traveled to Hong Kong to be a fit model for Calvin Klein Knitwear. This was my first trip to China. A friend of mine was a design director for Calvin Klein and she set me up with the gig. At the time, I just happened to be the right measurements for a male Calvin Klein fit model. Naturally, I had more Calvin Klein cashmere sweaters than anyone could dream of.

We stayed at the Mandarin Oriental hotel on Hong Kong Island. They have these lovely scented Hermés soaps and products in the rooms. I've always been a fan of the orange color of the Hermés branding, but not because it's attention getting.

Orange is a color I love. I find I am naturally drawn to it. Orange also happens to be the color of monk's robes and in some cultures considered to be auspicious. Color is a very important component of our psychology.

The Calvin Klein factories, at the time, were just a short ride from Hong Kong into China by train. For me this trip was a precursor to a career in tea. I always had an obsession with tea. Something about it was attractive to me, sexy even. I started drinking black coffee at nine years old. On New Year's Eve when I was 17 I drank so much Dunkin' Donuts coffee (light and sweet) I threw up in a parking lot as the new year rang in. After that I'd had my fill of drinking coffee and have drunk tea regularly since.

The Tea Shop Where It All Began

On our day off, my friend and I traveled almost all the way up to the top of the hill on Hong Kong Island. Where she had wanted to visit a tea shop. My friend was Chinese, and had grown up in Hong Kong. She had been to this tea shop many times before. A woman named Rose was the purveyor of the shop. They were speaking Cantonese, I sat and watched.

Rose was the ninth generation owner of this shop, and was over eighty years old. On that sunny afternoon we sat for many hours, tasting different teas. With each tea, Rose performed a ritual. Every tea had a story of origin, a story of process, a story of medicinal properties. Now and then my friend would translate some of these details.

On the walls were miniature drawers, about a thousand, all filled with varieties of tea. After we left I felt quite buzzed on caffeine. I'll never forget this experience. The way the hot afternoon sun shone at that angle, reflecting brightly off of the tea shop's sign. Ever since that experience I have gone on to consume tea, and learn as much about it as I could. By working in and brewing tea, I had an awakening.

Tea's Allegory For Humanity

Tea could tell the story of human civilization. Being the world's second most-consumed beverage, only bested by the main ingredient used to brew it, water. A simple shrub living for thousands of years. When consumed, it stimulates creation, conversation, and thought. Harvested and consumed by humans for five millennia.

The origin of tea has a wonderful birth legend. Tea leaves float on a breeze into an emperor's cup. Quite poetic prose. Today, tea is still an integral part of human history. Tea is also a very good allegory for humanity.

Over thousands of years tea has participated in countless political acts, dynasties, businesses, geopolitical affairs, wars, acts of espionage, dramatic and climactic storylines. Tea is a witness to human history and tells a long and compelling story. The chronicles a collective cup of tea would tell, if it were to speak, could only rival the stories shared by people over a pot of tea.

Herein is where I place my first dot, from tea to humans. Before there were telephones and the internet, there were messengers and scrolls. Whose stories were undoubtedly discussed many times over tea. Tea has been a true witness to history's greatest events, observing and participating in real time.

Tea Ceremony

In brewing tea, there is a saying: "to honor the tea," to respect and treat the leaves a certain way. Rose, who ran the tea shop in Hong Kong, honored the tea. Each time before she brewed tea, Rose would move her hand in a rhythmic and ceremonial way over the pot and cup. As if she was cleaning the spirit of past brews.

Before adding fresh leaves, she would pour hot water into the pot to rinse and warm the pot. Then she would add the leaves with a small amount of hot water to rinse the tea. After discarding the water a second time, she would add water a third time actually brewing the tea.

I could tell she had great regard and prized each leaf. During her ceremony she would tell the story of the tea leaves. What the flavor profile and medicinal properties may be. Which region the tea originated from, and how it was grown.

Over her lifetime she had probably done this same ritual more than a million times. In my opinion, tea is magical. As with all things magical, tea originally was only available to the wealthy and elite. Tea even served as currency before becoming available to the masses.

The stories tea has to share could never have been kept for only the select few. Since tea itself has a peculiar way of democratizing a situation. When people sit at a table to drink a cup, no matter their rank in life, they are at an equal level.

Pouring and sipping, a dialog ensues. Compelled by the tea to tell stories, to share ideas, and to bridge the gap. Warm, stimulating and comforting, tea uplifts our soul and enhances our mind. With the power to heal us physically and stimulate creativity, tea is humanity's energetic string throughout history. When past time returns.

Each Tea's Story Is Unique

To coax a story from tea is not hard. Yet, to hear all the notes and understand the prose fully does require a love for tea and a small amount of knowledge. Each harvest, season, region and so forth is unique.

Here is where I draw my allegory. The same could be said for humanity. Our roots, nourishment, mentors, education, season, enrichment, environment, experiences, thoughts, shape us no differently than the weather, region, soil, altitude, care, genes, health and artisans shape a tender, freshly picked green bud into the myriad of configurations, profiles and varieties of tea available today.

There are many factors that lead to a proper cup of tea. Like the season, geography, water, and weather. The artisans play an equally important role in the development of flavor profiles and quality of tea.

Not all tea leaves are created equally. Some are bitter, some bright, some fruity and some malty. Dark, light, yellow, black and green. Physically appearing: heavy, light, thick, thin, precious, soft, brittle and hard.

Many tea gardens are not sprayed with fertilizers, chemicals or even watered, except by the rain. Though they could be considered organic, in the modern sense, many are not certified. These shrubs live simply as they have been living. Long before conventional fertilizers came into being. Old growth trees, growing naturally as they have for hundreds, and some, for thousands of years.

Similar to wine (and humans) the terrain, environment and weather create individual characteristics and profiles, as does the altitude. Using a diverse array of techniques like shading, harvesting methods, heat, oxidation, fermentation, and aging. Artisans coax out the complexity and flavor notes from the still growing and freshly picked green leaves.

There is a very high level of skill and labor involved in processing tea. Most knowledge is generational, passed on through apprenticeships. Simply popping a bag with crushed, dried leaves in some hot water doesn't tell much of the story behind the leaf. Rather this leaf's story has been consumed by the brand. The energy in this style of tea has been commodified. Like tea, so have humans been commodified.

CHAPTER TWO

Modernity

As a child we fantasize about what we want to be when we grow up. We want to be someone with purpose. Then life comes along and molds us into shape and says be realistic, get an education, get a job, pay your bills, have a nice something-something, raise kids, find somewhere to live. Tending to follow the path set for us. Ask your parents, "Why do we do things this way?" You probably will get an answer something like, "Because that's the way things are done."

Some will say God tells us what to do, quoting stories from books. Written during a time when most humans did not know much about what was going on, or why they were, where they were. It's just how things are I imagine them thinking. Same as today. The thing with books of this sort is that they only tell stories, left to interpretation.

There is justification to this devotion in the belief that. "These words were passed down to us by a divine power." Yet, we will never know the true motivations of the writers, or the scribes. In all reality we can't. Nor, can we trust who actually dictated these words and for what purpose. There was a lot of interpretation going on back then.

Of course there's lots of theories and I don't aim to discredit them. Just prove a point about knowledge. In this type of situation. We will never truly be able to know the actual events. Because stories are after all, stories. And only can be what we are told, or has been written.

It's Our Programming

It's less thoughtful to follow and not question or think too much. Don't rock the boat, do what everyone else is doing, we resist conflict. Biologically, we are programmed this way. While for thousands of years religions have ruled the planet through the insistence of dogma and unquestioning loyalty. It might sound like a familiar tactic to us presently.

For millennia humans were forced to conform or be labeled as heretics. It's part of our collective psyche. Still to the present day we are conforming, fitting neatly into a box. Only now, we are conforming to being mass produced consumers. Like products on an assembly line. The producers make sure the followers stay within the lines, stop at the right stations, get the right attachments, firmware, applications and so forth.

If you think about an assembly line. Separating yourself from the usual, the required and scheduled stops. Deviating from the "correct" way of assemblage is a recipe for disaster.

How many times have you participated in an activity, or claimed to like something, acted in a certain way, solely because others did? Regardless of whether you personally wanted to participate, liked the activity, or wanted to act that way. Regardless of whether you truly agreed, as those around you seemed to. Probably when you start thinking about it you see you do it all the time. We all do it, that's why it's called groupthink.

Fear, Groupthink And Chemicals Manipulate Decision Making

Fear chemicals and decision making are a part of our daily life. Being objective and gaining an understanding of these processes will greatly improve our quality of life. We are such a funny species.

We are so adaptable, precisely why questioning the paradigm is difficult. We adapt to fit into social situations. Finding ourselves often making decisions and taking actions specifically because we are resisting conflict, because subconsciously we fear conflict. Or because we want to fit in.

When you take into consideration the control this fear wields on us every single day. Technically, you can only come to the conclusion that you are being controlled by fear. Simply because you don't know with certainty what another person's reaction will be. Or you don't want to "deal with it." We've all been there.

Psychologically we want to protect your own self image. But what you may not know is that food, chemicals and many other components are affecting these thoughts and decisions as well. It's much easier to control the fear of groupthink when you have the confidence and consciousness of a clear mind.

What If It's As Simple As Learning About Ourselves

Throughout this book I lay out a series of actions, scientific arguments and philosophies for your consideration. I draw from my experiences working in advertising, my time spent owning a health and wellness brand. And my own personal experiences spent researching foods and all things scientific regarding the gut..

I realized it was important to me to understand how all of these seemingly innocuous chemicals and manipulations affected my wellbeing. After many years living the lifestyle I detail in this book. I want to share what I have learned and am able to see clear as day. I think these ideas are important for everyone to consider in order for humans collectively to change our trajectory. To return us, dare I say, from the brink of self destruction. A dare of sorts to become "clean," or back to natural as I prefer to call it. To create a Living Environment for all.

Fear And Chemicals

Not only are there many chemicals in our food, air and water that are emotionally and micro-critically swaying our thoughts and actions every day. Humans, generally speaking, are wired to be afraid of the unknown.

It is important to come to a place where we can relate to and understand ourselves. We all have thoughts, cravings and fears. Understanding where each of these comes from, and analyzing why we have them, is a first important step in learning about ourselves.

Manipulating The World Around Us To Fit Our Perspective

For the last few hundred years plus, rather than bending to, and integrating with the world around us, humans have taken a hard edged, top down approach. We are the alpha species, taking the natural world, manipulating, and commodifying it. Claiming ownership of it for ourselves and for profit. Before modernity and industrialization people needed to rely on the natural world. There was still a connection to the rhythms of nature.

Part of the human experience is a sense of territorialism, as with all animals there is an innate sense to lay claim to, and defend what we perceive to be ours. This leads us to fear outsiders because the outsider is an unknown who might lay claim to our claim.

For an easy example, there are many cases of a black man walking in a white neighborhood, with a perfectly good reason to be there. Yet, someone invariably calls the police, or worse assaults the black man. You might say he doesn't blend in. Simply because of his color he stands out.

The same as a white person does in a predominantly black neighborhood. This behavior is rooted deep in our DNA. We seek out breaks in patterns. Mentally and physically, humans are consciously and subconsciously landscaping territories individually, collectively, and tribally.

A Break In The Connection To The Natural World

Our modern existence has caused a break in connection to the natural world. Instead of integrating with it, the human species is tearing the natural world apart and reassembling it from shards like a puzzle with no defined picture, besides a profit sign.

We are bending everything around us to meet our demands, our point of view, our selfish and unnecessary physical needs and our thoughts of how things "should be." Manipulating everything, even reality.

This way of reasoning has caused us to lose touch with the energy and love for nature. Throwing things out of balance. We begin to start missing that deep connection between our species and nature. For example, you can feel this connection when you go into the forest. It provides perspective, refreshes, calms and reconnects our sense of empathy.

Manipulation, Manifestation And Gaslighting

Three interesting words. Manipulation done in the proper way, through manifestation for the collective and self betterment, can be a good thing. Overall that doesn't seem to be happening though. Maybe using the term "gaslighting" is preferable to the idea I am trying to convey—we are gaslighting ourselves and others around us. It's time to change your reality.

Human survival is actually dependent on the collective. Egocentric selfishness is in part a product of advertising, manipulative messaging, and our consumeristic, consumption-based, endless economic growth paradigm. This paradigm uses humans like tools. Built for the sake of profits.

Re-Integrating With The Natural World

Many humans have come before us and integrated with the world around them. Inherent human adaptability and malleability is a blessing, and our curse. If we control our own malleability, using it to benefit our own personal development. We are able to mold ourselves to the collective benefit, we are in control.

However, when we secede this control to a greater power. We become the subjects and tools of those in power. Packed neat and tidy, molded into conformity. Manipulated to consume, we do as we are told for fear of rocking the boat.

My Personal Epiphany

My reason for writing this book. For one, it's cathartic for me. I had an epiphany. I was just like everyone else. One day I woke up and I just couldn't take part in the endless negativity and destruction anymore. I had come to a point where I became overtly aware of the damage being done to the planet, our physical bodies and our energetic consciousness. It had all become too great for me. I was overloaded. And I needed to reset my circuit.

I strongly believe the only product we should be considering is ourselves. How you personally reflect on those and the world around you. We need to ask ourselves everyday: Are my actions benefiting or negating our environment? How about your best "self" and those around you? Do you really need all the possessions in your life? Is one-upping your neighbor or friend really worth the negative ripples? Do you think generating endless amounts of waste will never add up?

What Is Truly Our Purpose?

For me, this life is about gaining wisdom for our energetic consciousness. It's not about being a wage or debt slave so I can consume everything that tickles my fancy. Even if I was very wealthy. I would still live relatively simply. I am not a collector of things. For the weight can be great.

Once you are able to separate yourself from the upside-down paradigm. And are able to turn yourself right side up. You see more clearly the ways in which you are being manipulated every day by your food, chemicals, advertising and those in power.

Throughout this book I reference dozens of scientific studies and cite many personal examples from my life. This information helped bring about the realizations for me. Our diets and systems are so unbelievably upside-down. I urge you to break free, and take control of your own quality of life and your children's. Take real, actual control. Recognize the subtleties of how your thoughts are influenced every minute, of every day. Gain the power to block out all of the toxins, messaging and resist the cravings.

Seeing The Picture Clearly

My aim is to tie a multitude of seemingly disparate information together. Like individual puzzle pieces, I assemble this information into a clear picture and narrative. How the food we eat, advertising and our political systems shape who we are as energetic beings in our current epoch, the Anthropocene. Even though recently the panel that decides the naming convention for these types of things rejected calling our period the Anthropocene. I will continue to refer to it in this book for the sake of consistency.

It's time to take the red pill and wake up. There is no way to be objective of this reality, if there is no way to compare it to a different reality. There is, however, another reality right here. Right inside of you.

You hold it, you possess it, it is yours to control. But you have to snap out of the fake world and see it. It's not as dystopian as in The Matrix. It's actually more fantastic than the reality we live in now. But if humans collectively can't move out of this fever dream we live in, it is possible it may slip away for good.

CHAPTER THREE

Culture

Culture is a very broad and potentially dangerous category to discuss. Strong opinions exist here. When I reference culture my emphasis is on recognizing cultural norms that are stifling yours, and humanity's evolution to be our best selves. Cultural norms are being used against us as whips. Inhibiting people from being their best selves. Eating, acting, living in a way that our current "culture" dictates for us.

Many times culture involves conserving familiar ways of doing something, languages and ideas from the past. Often though, culture is as simple as staying up to date with what is current on TV. Or having the latest whatever it is everyone in your peer group has, or is talking about.

Social Culture

One example is water cooler talk at the office about the latest TV show or movie. If you don't watch TV or if you are not up to date with the latest episode. Then you won't understand the references. Maybe you won't feel like you fit in, and it's possible your peers will make fun of you.

If you are not on social media or if you don't have the newest sneakers like your peers, the latest piece of technology, or whatever it is that your peer group is doing. You may feel left out and suffer from "FOMO," fear of missing out. Fear is the hook and line of social grouping and culture. Humans have an endless need to feel they "fit in."

The Human Algorithm

In my opinion, this is a purposeful defect in the human algorithm. Like a back door for a hacker, this defect is being exploited and used to keep us in check. Through advertising and by manipulating the weakest links. This keeps us chasing consumption based ideologies, trying to fit in and be like everyone else. Because fitting in, is doing what everyone else is doing.

If you are able to feel confident in who you are individually, then you may not find yourself in the position of needing to be like everyone else. This feeling of confidence comes with mental strength, self awareness and acceptance of yourself. But I also believe it's necessary to bring yourself back to "natural" to find this happy place. By eliminating the outside influences and toxins. You will rewrite your own algorithm. Because that is how the human brain and artificial intelligence works.

In this "happy place" your personality is not being pushed or pulled by inside or outside forces. You control your thoughts and recognize your decision making and emotions. You become in touch with the ways each piece is being influenced.

After making the mental switch. Recognizing certain types of culture and possessions are weaknesses. Weights that are holding you back. Manipulating you to live and act in a certain way. Ways that are not efficient or beneficial to your quality of life. You may become determined not to let yourself be manipulated again.

Maybe I am only speaking for myself, but I think probably not. I don't like to be manipulated, especially against my own best interests. I don't actually feel left out. It's quite the opposite, I feel freer than ever. Sure at first it was hard. But nothing worth doing is easy right? Taking this power back. Will empower you.

And let me state that I don't mean to say all forms of culture are bad. I am simply trying to convey that culture is a means of power wielded over us. It is important to note the difference. Preserving a cultural dance is not the same as buying presents for Christmas. One is built from artistic expression. The other however, is built as a commodified expression, based in consumerism.

The Truth About American Christmas' Culture Of Gift Giving

When giving became taking and spun as giving. Once again a story emerges where those in power take from those less fortunate. In his book, The Battle for Christmas, historian Stephen Nissenbaum explains how the consumerist expression of Christmas came about.

Starting in New York City in the Early 1800s. Elites waged a campaign to move the holiday celebrations out of the streets and into the homes of the working poor. As it was customary during this time period for the poor to ask the elites for food and drinks while celebrating outdoors. Simultaneously, there was a new growing middle class in NYC. These parents wished to "keep their children safe at home." While also introducing them, on their terms, to take part in the new rise of commercial products.

It's an interesting story. And it begs asking. What are traditions? Is it familiarity and routine? I mean who doesn't love Christmas? Someone say vacation? Probably, that is one piece of the puzzle. Digging deeper another story emerges about who is truly benefiting most? Think about it, it's a brilliant system.

Culture Often Isn't Healthy

There are many cultural foods and behaviors that are just plain bad for our health. Many popular modern cultural expressions are just not healthy for society. Like the idolization of celebrities or the rich. I am sure you must be familiar with some foods and culture you grew up with. That when looked at from an objective point of view, might be recognized as not healthy.

For example why do humans place so much importance on water cooler talk about a TV show? One angle, it is a way to bond with work mates. Yet, often TV shows depict actions that are meant to keep us distracted or introduce us to ideas. While enforcing negative cultural or stereotypical behaviors and the status quo. Because humans want to fit in and are searching for approval. They begin to act out these situations. This system is used against us and we keep reinforcing it. Making us weak and prone to manipulation.

Learn From History And Apply Those Lessons To Move Forward

There are many merited arguments in favor of preserving traditions and cultures. In my opinion, unfortunately many do not serve freedom of expression and are acting as means of control to hold us back. There are many reasons to learn from and cherish history. Yet, equally as many reasons to change, evolve and live in the present.

Have we not grown and learnt as humans since the past? Shouldn't we be applying lessons learned from the past by looking towards and moving into the future? Understanding why so much emphasis is placed on traditions and preserving cultural norms. As an arm of our current "culture wars." Will help to understand exactly how these ways of being are holding humanity back, and are being used against us.

Routine Is Easy, Breaking Routine Is Hard

Familiarity and repetition are easy. The human animal seems to crave routine. Doing the same thing every day and acting like a machine. Maybe boring and easy is good. Change is very hard for many to accept and accepting yourself, and your faults, is even harder. Yet, it is extremely powerful and fulfilling. However, changing requires effort. It also can mean going against the grain.

Many of us are already overworked, over stressed, and overly polluted. By taking the chance to change your reality. Ultimately, what do you have to lose? You may learn something very rewarding about yourself. Recognizing positive and negative cultural aspects is part of critical thinking. Changing is part of evolution. Look at our natural history. Animals evolve and evolve and so forth.

Sometimes humans do question the paradigm. But more often than not, they go right back to living in it, within seconds of questioning it. Questioning cultural norms and asking: "Why do we do these things when really they serve us no benefit?" And then actually following through on our diagnosis. Means doing something different. Which is a recipe to be penalized or ostracized. It seems without escape.

When do we get to be our true selves living free from the manipulative effects of society? The system is built upside-down to keep us this way. Repeating the same things over and over removes the fear. Fear of what lies ahead of us. The unknown is a risk. Humans like familiar and easy. Risk of the unknown is hardwired into our brain to be "bad." Today is a fantastic day to break free and embrace the unknown.

CHAPTER FOUR

Size & Scale

There is a microbiome story line running parallel to our human lives. One of living relationships, nature, understanding, connectedness, and codependency. It's very possible that what we cannot see is of more importance, and influence on us, than that which can be seen.

Are We An Avatar?

What if we consider the idea that the human body is an avatar? Because really, we are avatars in more ways than one. Humans could be said to be an avatar for the soul or energetic spirit. Or, in this life, humans could simply be players in a game for an advanced dimensional species. Humans could even be avatars for microscopic aliens. No one really can answer with certainty why we are here. An unknown unknown.

Here is where kombucha comes back into focus. Humans are literally walking, talking biofilms. Another word used to describe a biofilm is SCOBY, which stands for a Symbiotic Culture Of Bacterias and Yeasts. This description is used in kombucha brewing. The SCOBY is what grows on top of the fermenting tea. Protecting it from invaders and contamination. The SCOBY is a hotel of sorts. This term could also be used loosely to describe the human body.

We Are More Invisible Organisms Than Visible Ones

Some scientists have calculated that the human body is made up of more microbiota (57%) than cellular structure (43%) with the greatest concentration of microbiota in the bowel. "They are essential to your health," says Professor Ruth Ley, the director of the department of microbiome science at the Max Planck Institute. "Your body isn't just you." Not only that, the genes of these microbiota could outnumber our human DNA by as much as 1000:1—this means we have to consider that we are more than simply "our" human DNA.

Professor Rob Knight, from the University of California San Diego, has done some experiments on mice. These mice were born into a world completely free of microbes. What he found is incredible. He says: "We were able to show that if you take lean and obese humans and take their feces and transplant the bacteria into mice you can make the mouse thinner or fatter depending on whose microbiome it got." Could you imagine the diet pills?! Well you don't have to. Because this type of therapy exists for humans. With the same results.

Our Microbiome Is Kinda Like A Pet

We don't know what we don't know. It behooves us to treat our bodies with the utmost respect, love, and attention. Because it may very well be that our lives are dependent on the wellness of our microbiome and the relationships we have with our microbiota.

In this situation our personal wellness becomes a function of the quality of our relationships. Not only with our friends, family, and peers, but also with the unseen world. The quality of our relationships is a function of the quality of our wellness...and so it goes. It's a microcosm of the macrocosm.

Whether we like it or not, whether we acknowledge it or not. Our lives are dependent on our relationship with bacteria, yeasts, fungi and archaea living on and inside of our bodies. The best thing we can do is try to nurture them like pets or guard dogs. At least the good ones!

Checking Into The SCOBY Hotel

Humans could be said to be a SCOBYFA, since we would add in Fungi and Archaea. Technically speaking, yeasts are a subsection of fungi, more about this later. Archaea are prokaryotes, single celled organisms that lack a nucleus and other membrane-bound organelles. The science here is very fascinating.

We humans are quite literally a hotel, housing more microbiota and genes than our own cellular structure and genes. These bacteria, yeasts, archaea, and fungi live inside our body as well as on the outside. They are everywhere. They control and mitigate some of the functionality of our bodies—more than we know.

Where Do They All Come From

The scientific community really doesn't know where bacteria come from. And we are just barely beginning to learn how important they are to our health. As a fan of science fiction, I have created a Sci-Fi story to illustrate a point. Plus, it's a weird story to read before I get into the more heavy stuff to come. Take a trip down into the rabbit hole. Imagine we exist solely to feed and shelter these guests.

Our "body" is a living biofilm, a SCOBYFA controlled by aliens. Human's could be the living bio-robots of an advanced alien race. Never even knowing it. Maybe more than one alien race. A galaxy's worth, competing for control, literally and metaphorically, right under our noses. Forget the Lizard People. Watch out for the Probiotic Pirates.

Here Come The Probiotic Pirates

Three billion years ago. Millions of light years away. An explosion hurtled a comet made of ice and minerals through the black, vast, cold expanse of space. Set on a collision course with Earth and trapped in the ice—Transcdecent tea and Probiotic Pirates. How did the probiotic pirates get here? They would ask themselves if they could, "When were we frozen solid." But, no one was coherent at this time to ponder such an occurrence.

It wasn't always this way in their home world. The probiotic pirates were just like everyone else, all million, zillion, billion, trillion, quadrillion of them. Pirating in the sweet, temperate freshwater seas of Meet Lamd. The planetary database labels sector MEET, co-ordinate, MtLN3D. Colloquially known as Meet Lamd. A planet with very shallow seas which covers precisely 57%.

Welcome To Meet Lamd

Geographically speaking, the Mount Everest of Meet Lamd would be an easy hike up to 3.1 meters above sea level. Except that you could never walk on Meet Lamd. Over the other 43% grows a sugary sweet, sticky vegetation which has fat, hollow, gelatinous stalks and very spiky branches. The vegetation is known simply in English as Sticky plant. Occupying a unique place in the evolution of this planet. Sticky plant is the only known vegetation growing on this planet.

Sticky plant especially thrives when growing near geothermal vents where a unique mineral composition gives vitality to the plant. Its leaves harvest luminescence from Meet Lamd's three suns each one a different age, warmth, distance, and orbit. All shine in varying wavelengths of light, feeding the most deeply saturated, iridescent sticky plant leaves.

It's A Stubby Little Fat Spiky Tree

Like a stubby tree, sticky plant grows in a wide spherical-coned, volcano like structure upwards toward this sector's suns. Erupting, oozing, and spurting a very sweet, sticky, sucrose like substance as it grows. Eventually, the outside membrane hardens like a bark.

When sticky plant grows above the high tide levels, icicle shaped branches sprout outward. At the very tip of each icicle like limb grows eight, perfect, octagon shaped, baseball sized leaves.

Like translucent solar panels they glitter and shimmer a laser-bathed, velour textured disco ball of reflected light. They are quite a treat for the receptors of species which are able to see in broad wavelengths of light. The whole planet itself is rather remarkable, in its weirdness.

Erupting, Oozing Disco Balls - But No Partying Allowed

The leaves, having never been scientifically studied, thrive using what is suspected to be a peculiar process. Giving life to this very strange plant, which appears to be creating significantly more sugars and starches than needed. Hence, all the erupting and oozing.

Advanced species nearby watch Meet Lamd through their telescopes. The glittery, rainbow disco ball of a planet doesn't shoot stars. Instead, it shoots disco ball beams of light wavelengths onto nearby worlds. Refracted from the sticky plant's leaves.

Meet Lamd does not allow tourists. Not that there is a sign or a government. It's more of a general warning in this sector. When you punch an address into the map quest guidance of your starship, a pop up tab warns of known celestial bodies to avoid in each sector due to certain unforgiving conditions.

Like the bugs on AXXXXXZ99, they will eat you. One time there was a glitch in the map quest guidance system and the pop up blocker became enabled for all users. What a political drama.

Speaking of politics. There is no immigration bureau on Meet Lamd. Advanced species have been known to visit. Even some attempt refuge. Those with the capabilities to breach the atmosphere on Meet Lamd must wear special goggles. Or be blinded by the refracted light from the sticky plant leaves.

The Only Being Ever Known To Live On Meet Lamd

One famous star junk pirate, John Henry Mathew, an outlaw from the Cyprus moons. Who is said to be guilty of crimes against his shipmates. Is rumored to have successfully survived on Meet Lamd for three Earth months. The trick is, he is rumored to have said, "Never land yourself on, well, land." Land is a soggy, sticky, spiky bog. That literally has you stuck there, blinded and impaled. In that spot. Forever.

Just Your Typical Solar System

Like all solar systems, the suns and nearby moons push and pull the seas and vegetation. The closest, and hottest star—named JUNK17 because of its high elliptical orbit—moves at a very high velocity.

This star gives Meet Lamd seasons of exactly 31 days. In the hot season, the younger, top layers of the sticky plant wither. The plant senses this and immediately discards the leaves. These leaves then become stuck around the base of the trees where they ferment.

Around the same time, moon JACKO3 coincides its orbit. Every moon orbiting every planet is named JackO and given a number designation. This is what happens when you let children of politicians give celestial bodies names.

The gravitational effects of both the sun and the moon cause the tides and magma below the surface to rise. Hot magma underneath the surface of the Meet Lamd regularly heats the surrounding vicinity high tides up to 2.1 times the normal temperature of 88 degrees Fahrenheit. The heated water readily dissolves the sticky sugars. While this is happening, the sticky plant leaves steep into a very beautiful, hibiscus hued tea. That also happens to have a lovely orange-violet-esq, iridescent shimmer.

Just Sticky Plant And The Microbes

On this world, all the plants produce this sugar-like substance because all the plants are sticky plant. This is a planet of microscopic life thriving on sugars and starches. There is one species that has evolved and even could be considered a dominant mammal species on this planet. However, it did not begin its existence here. Supposedly, it was imported by none other than John Henry Mathew.

Yet, it did evolve rather quickly since it has no natural predators on Meet Lamd. The Mookie Wuuk, something like a duck, is food for many species in this sector. A mammal that floats in shallow seas or other bodies of water.

The Mookie Wuuk

The Mookie Wuuk go where the tide takes them, feeding and getting around using techniques which could be attributed to a wood-pecker, ant-eater, sail-boat. But don't be confused by the description. The size of the Mokkie Wuuk is about that of an oversized Earth chicken. It uses its hairless, large, heart shaped tail as a rudder, oar, and sail.

To feed the Mookie Wuuk uses its snout to bore holes through the outer crust of sticky plant trunks. This allows sticky plant tea to seep inside and ferment. The Mookie Wuuk then insert their long symmetrically grooved tongue. With a texture somewhat like a cat's tongue. It slurps sticky plant juice, sticky plant tea, and the meat of the plant. Kinda like a fermenty, meaty Boba Tea, but without all the branding.

The end of its tongue has a little set of spiky, snakelike teeth. Which the Mookie Wuuk uses to hollow out sticky plant meat lining the inside of the plants trunk, much like the inside of a coconut. Eventually the sticky plant will die because of all this and break in half, leaving a solid, hollow outer shell. Something like a tree stump sized version of a caldera.

As with any food chain, the Mookie Wuuk has grown to serve a role for the probiotic pirates. Mookie Wuuk feeding causes the sticky plant trees to weaken, break, and collapse, leaving a hollow stump behind.

When the tides rise, these hollow stumps fill with sweetened, heated, and steeped transcdecent tea. Named so by John Henry Mathew. He said when you drink it you are able to transcend dimensionality. Whatever that means. When the tides recede, the remaining sticky plant tea remains inside the hollow stump fermenting. Resulting in an explosion of Probiotic Pirates and all other cohorts of microbiota.

Birthday Party!

When a female Mookie Wuuk is ready to give birth. She will remain floating in the caldera of a broken sticky plant tree. After the tides recede, she will give birth inside these transcdecent tea pools full of probiotic Pirates.

The newborns, having already been fed sticky transcdecent tea in the womb, are born with a love (addiction) for slurping the sweet fermented sticky plant tea. This offers the Probiotic Pirates fresh real estate to colonize inside the digestive system of the baby Mookie Wuuks. There they will set up and live inside the Mookie Wuuk's gut. Sending signals to the brain to eat and slurp more fermented transcdecent tea. And so the cycle repeats itself.

The newborns float off, with full bellies, on the next tide. With each excretion, they spread Probiotic Pirates into the surrounding waters. There they wait dormant. Dormant, that is, until the right conditions and food source awakens them.

CHAPTER FIVE

Knowledge

It's possible in some ways to see this book as hypocritical. For instance, if I say the only knowledge known. Is the knowledge which humans are taught or learned. Imagine uploaded data. In such cases there is not really any comparison. Meanwhile, I am writing this book using knowledge that is taught and learned. But there is at least a fig leaf here, science. Through comparisons scientists are able to perform experiments with quantifiable results.

We can't compare our existence on Earth to life on another planet or in another dimension. I have to use what is familiar to try to convey philosophical ideas, facts and theories. In this chapter I am going to talk about our knowledge system, lack thereof and energetic knowledge. In an attempt to stimulate the reader to think more creatively.

Starting where I left off in the previous chapter: the reason for the story about the probiotic pirates. It is labeled as a fictional story here in this book. But it is also just as possible that in the process of creating the idea, I created Meet Lamd in reality in some far off dimension or galaxy. It is also equally probable that bacteria on Earth arrived from a meteor, from another galaxy, or even from another dimension. The truth is, no one really knows.

The Invisible Microbiome Working For Us

Microorganisms form a very important role in the food chain and decomposition. In the soil they make nutrients available for plants.

Inside the human gut they do the same, making nutrients bioavailable for humans. These microbes are essential for life on this planet and proper gut health in humans. If they were to die out, so would humans.

In the last decade, scientists have only begun to learn how different bacterial compositions are within our gut. And how these compositions change the function of our brain, health and bodies, by altering our perception, mood, well-being, genes, and cognitive abilities. They have even been found to cause strokes. This is amazing breakthrough science of which we have only just scratched the surface.

Yeasts, fungi and bacteria are different in every city, town, and home worldwide. Why are there so many different species of yeasts, fungi, archaea, and bacteria living in our bodies and everywhere around us? Where do these microorganisms come from?

Scientists have a theory. About three billion years or so ago they may have formed in the seas or maybe they rained down from the skies. However, these same scientists admit that no one truly knows where bacteria came from. It is very important to absorb this concept about our knowledge.

Do We Really Know Anything?

Contrary to contemporary egocentric beliefs, human knowledge in this physical form is quite insignificant. Ultimately, we really have no idea how we came to be. Sure there is the theory of evolution. It is a valid theory. But one has to accept there could be many other theories as well.

Did aliens come to Earth and splice monkeys with their DNA? Is this all just a holographic simulation? What if all the evidence we find, buried in the Earth, was planted there for us to find? Maybe everything we think we know is a total set up and manipulation like a video game.

Our History Of Truth In Knowledge

When we look back into history and review humanities teachings, or medicines, for example. You find that in each era, there are ideas, teachings or theories presented as "truths." However, with time, many of those truths have been found to be untrue. Let's keep this in mind when contemplating the truths of our current era.

Philosophy Meets Science

French philosopher Alain Badiou argues that truth is a witnessed event. Constructed through process. The process being, the witnessing of said event. By witnessing it and naming it into worldly situations we write its "truth." He argues that ontology is situational. Meaning that every person's existence is based on their situation. Each individual's experience of a situation is how they view the truth of the world.

Further, since we cannot account for, or know all situations. That which we know as truth, or in the case here, knowledge. Is only what we experience it as, an "event" or "situation." Meaning the only truth we know is from what we are experiencing. Our experiences of life here and now. Caught up in the minutia of the day to day.

Regardless of what was "learned" or "experienced." In my view, humanity mostly has no idea what is going on. The knowledge we know, mostly comes without comparison. No matter what you think, study, learn or believe. We cannot put human existence in any context. There is no comparison.

Therefore, how could we truly have an objective understanding of why or how we got here. Or what our existence is, in comparison to other intelligent life forms. Of course we can feel like it's this or that reason. Humans can make up theories and study so called evidence. But we can't even be sure if the physical world we live in is real. And many credible scientists seem to agree, it's not real!

These same scientists theorize that, in fact, this world is not real, and more of a simulation or hologram instead. Ultimately, we are just hurtling through space, counting what we call time, on what we believe to be a rock. A human named Earth. Living in what I like to call the "stone age" of an idea we express as "technological advancement."

The Quantum Mechanics World View

Let's get a bit technical. Quantum mechanics is a very fascinating field of study. The quantum model of physics states that the physical world is 99.99999% energy and .00001% matter, meaning atoms are mostly empty space and fields of energy.

Very briefly I majored in Chemical Engineering at Northeastern University in Boston and absolutely love physics and chemistry, but was not good enough at engineering math. Even though I never came close to completing my studies at Northeastern. I still do my best to read up on the latest advancements in theoretical physics.

When I began to learn about quantum theory, it just blew my mind. The key to remember with quantum mechanics is that the electron of the atom does not appear in a position until you view it. This is called "manifesting the wavelength," or "collapsing the wave function."

A bit like what I think Alain Badiou means when we witness an event we record it as truth. Once witnessed, at that point the electron appears as a particle in position. This could simply be interpreted that by thinking and viewing, we are creating. Quantum mechanics is the secret to manifesting humanity's future selves and makes good sense of the theory that this life is actually a simulation.

If This Is All A Simulation What Can We Do About It?

You are probably wondering what gut health and quantum mechanics have to do with each other. Here is how I see it. Quantum mechanics rules the world we live in. Energy is a very important aspect of the world of quantum mechanics. There are scientific studies which show that by controlling our personal energy, humans are able to use that energetic focus to manipulate statistical outcomes and DNA strands simply with thoughts. So it would seem quantum mechanics has a lot more to do with things than we can perceive.

The Gut Brain Connection

Studies have shown that bacteria in our gut affect our mood, cognitive abilities, well-being and so on. This is why gut health is so important. If we accept that our world view is dictated by the microbiome living in our gut. We must also recognize that if our mood is dour and the cause is poor gut health, or poor diet. This affects the body's ability to metabolize nutrients amongst a host of negative side effects.

We all know that when we are grumpy from a sugar crash, hangover, or because we are hungry. That our energy signature and brain function isn't the same as when we are operating at 100%. This in turn affects our ability to be our best selves and use our energy to manifest positive situations.

Remember with quantum mechanics it is all about manifesting the wavelength. Meaning that if we focus hard enough building a picture in our mind and our energy is congruent with the quantum field that surrounds everything. Then we can bring that idea into reality. If we all have negative voices in our head this steers the manifestation of situations into a different direction. When you eliminate the voices by detoxifying your body and changing your inputs. Steering the ship in a positive way becomes a piece of cake.

When our energy signature is not congruent this can leave us stuck or going in circles. Imagine your body is like a formula one race car and you keep putting cheap gasoline in the tank. This is how your gut health and the gut brain connection work together with energy to steer each individual's reality.

What If Gut Health Affects Quantum Mechanics Through Decision Making

A major part of your personal system is decision making and its ripple effect. If you replay past events in your life. You will find jumping off points that lead you in one direction, or another. Most people probably don't realize that every daily decision you make in your life has a ripple effect. If I never drank that bottle of kombucha I never would have written this book.

For example, maybe there's a great networking event. If your gut health is poor and you are afraid that you might have to run to the bathroom at this event and you don't like public toilets. You may choose to skip the event all together. In turn missing an opportunity. One that was meant to be there for you. You will never know how this one event could have changed your life.

But there are also many more subtle ways that gut health can affect your decision making process and you won't even know it. It's these very subtle manipulations that are actually not so subtle when they add up. In the end only you are responsible for your decisions and your health. The best you can do to keep your energy congruent with the quantum field is to make sure that you have great gut health and maintain healthy gut brain connection. Think of your body like an antenna. Depending on the type of bacteria in your gut the signal will change. They don't call your gut your second brain for nothing!

Everything Is Energy And Nothing Is Matter

Another key point to take away here is that everything is energy. Specifically, 99.9999% energy and only .00001% matter. The physical world only seems real to us because of electromagnetic forces and wave functions. I think maybe it is not the easiest concept to fully grasp. Energy is an opportunity waiting to happen.

According to Ali Sundermier who works as a Science Communications Officer at the US Department of Energy. "Since the meat of your atoms is nestled away in nuclei, when you 'touch' someone (or something), you aren't actually feeling their atoms. What you're feeling is the electromagnetic force of your electrons pushing away their electrons. On a very, very technical level, you're not actually sitting on that chair. You're hovering ever so slightly above it. So to conclude: Your very important human body is really, kind of, in a way, just a misleading collection of empty spaces on an empty planet in an empty Universe." Yup, that about says it.

Accepting this will change your life. To use a cultural analogy, most people have probably seen Star Wars. When the characters talk about "The Force" this is kinda what I am talking about here. This is one thing quantum mechanics seeks to define. The force of energy that is in everything and how it operates.

Humans Are A Collection Of Sensors And Processors

Everyday humans are using processors and sensors, collecting information, parsing data, and writing reports. I am not talking about using computers. I mean our physical bodies. We have a multitude of sensors built right in.

Yes, humans created machines. In a way these machines aim to be replicants of humans to do the work humans have been doing. Yes, the singularity is coming. This is when computers become "smarter" when compared to humans. AI, artificial intelligence, is supposed to lead the way.

As of now, AI is just as biased and flailing as humanity. How could it not be since it is learning from and based on humanities knowledge? It too has no objective viewpoint from which to compare. Only the viewpoint given by its programmers and those from which it learns. AI learns only what is known already and then attempts to calculate beyond it. Even the researchers admit they do not know how it works.

Artificial Intelligence In Not The Greatness It's Made Out To Be

Although with Chat GPT and the recent advances in AI. Chat functions are improving. We can't forget situations like Microsoft's AI twitter bot Tay. Its Twitter profile read, "Tay is an artificial intelligent chat bot developed by Microsoft's Technology and Research and Bing teams to experiment with and conduct research on conversational understanding."

Tay only lasted 24 hours on Twitter, because it became so racist and offensive after "learning" from humans posting online. Be skeptical of AI. It is not the great breakthrough that the nine companies who are investing in it make it out to be. Five in the US and the rest of them are in China.

This includes facial recognition, which is also inherently racist. These things should concern all of us. Speaking at the Oslo Freedom Forum Jack Dorsey Twitter cofounder had this to say, "This is going to sound a little bit crazy, but I think the free speech debate is a complete distraction right now. I think the real debate should be about free will."

He went on "We are being *programmed*. We are being programmed based on what we say we're interested in, and we're told through these discovery mechanisms what is interesting—and as we engage and interact with this content, the algorithm continues to build more and more of this bias." Elon Musk chimed in, "Yeah, Jack is right."

In his view, even if an algorithm is open-source it's still opaque. Because it's not possible to predict or make models to show how it works and what the output will be at any given time and it can be changed at any time as well.

"Because people have become so dependent on it, it's actually changing and impacting the agency we have," Dorsey cautioned. "We can resist it all we want, but it knows us better than we know us, because we tell it our preferences implicitly and explicitly all the time, and it just feels super dangerous to continue to rely on that."

He saved the best part for last. "Five companies are building tools that we will all become entirely dependent upon," Dorsey said. "And because they're so complicated, we have no idea how to verify the correctness, we have no idea how to verify how they work, [or] what they're actually doing,"

Xenobots

Another recent and somewhat concerning development. In 2021 scientists built the world's first living robots, which are able to replicate. They call them "xenobots." Created from the cells of a frog. What's to say that humans are not already replicating artificial intelligence? We just can't know.

Robert Edward Grant

Speaking of cybernetics I'd like to introduce you to someone I find interesting. His name is Robert Edward Grant. I suggest any reader of this book visit his website and read some of his publications. He holds patents and various intellectual property in the fields of DNA and phenotypic expression, human cybernetic implantology, biophotonics, and electromagnetism with multiple publications in unified mathematics and physics.

I mention him because he has done some amazing tests using sound waves. The results imply that humans are made from binary code (zeros and ones) set into our DNA through frequencies. Frequencies make sense, because frequencies are wave functions. Quantum mechanics operates through the manifestation of waves. So how does an energetic consciousness come into being? By manifesting the waves (energy) into DNA apparently.

Other scientists have surmised we are living in a hologram. The multiverse, a Calabi-Yau manifold. . . and so forth. There are many theories as to what "this" is. What life on Earth is. What the meaning of life is. To think about it is human.

We Just Don't Know What Human Existence Is

One thing is for sure: Humans. Have. No. Idea. Hold onto this thought and don't forget it. Because this is one of humanity's main issues. Everyday humans go about their lives believing they know it all and are certain they are right. We are rightly over confident.

People will say, "I just feel it," "I just know it," or "it was written in a book or seen on TV." There are times when intuition can be, and is correct. Yet, to be brutally honest with ourselves is to recognize that humanity actually has no idea why humanity is here, what humanity is doing here, or why things are the way they are. Other than, this is how it was when we "lived." During the "Anthropocene." Of course there are naturally some things humans can and do measure. That can be and are proven.

But the big picture, the big why? Humanity just doesn't know. So we go about our days inventing things for the sake of making profits and trudge forward. Some of these inventions, ideas, and things are indeed good for humanity.

But many, probably the majority, are not. Humanity is just moving forward without a path or plan. Very often reliving past mistakes. Very easily sidetracked and distracted we lose focus. Like a goldfish in a bowl keeps swimming into the glass wall. We seem to keep forgetting we're trapped in a fishbowl.

Overconfidence Creates Problems

Everyday humans act with supreme confidence. Like we know what's going on. Going to work, school and learning. Taking comfort in our ideas and dissection of life. Yet, what a human learns as truth will be different from one part of the country and world to another.

Just look to China and Russia for examples. For an easy example their truth on the war in Ukraine and many other subjects won't match with that of the majority of others. So with the exception of math, math is truth. Truth in learning can be subjective. The majority of things that humans learn is only information which is fed to us. No different than uploading different data sets to a computer.

Our Personal Data Collection

Growing old, studying and exploring. Interacting with gravity and the natural world, the physical world. Each one of us develops hypotheses, theories, ideas, and conspiracies. Some of us test them. Some prove them. Others just know them to be true, they will say, without any evidence or proof.

Humanity has built machines and invented things to make life easier, to make living more convenient, and make tasks less time consuming. Just a few hundred years ago humans couldn't even be sure if the Earth was round. Even today, despite the vast photographic evidence from satellites and astronauts, some people still don't believe the Earth is round.

The Physics Of A Game Called Earth

On Earth we have what I like to call, the physics of a game called Earth. Gravity, Newtonian Physics and Relative Theory. They define the mechanics of our world and universe.

The Golden Ratio

Our natural world on this planet follows a very predictable formula called the Golden Ratio. A major component of the physics of a game called Earth. Some examples: the shape of a nautilus or snail shell, a hurricane, a spiral galaxy, human faces, flowers and DNA molecules. They all grow to fit within this ratio. Even stocks trade using it.

I find it compelling that there's such an order in our natural world. It lends credence, in my opinion, to the theory that this is all just a simulation. Imagine a video game. When a developer designs a video game, all of the mechanics have to follow certain rules and set parameters. These defined 'physics' make the outcomes predictable, allowing the characters to exist and interact within the game world with order and reliability.

Which Came First, Order Or Chaos

In some ways I think that the order of our world is an argument that it is not real. In a true "natural" world one might surmise everything would be random, not orderly. I think that UFO sightings and NDE's (Near Death Experiences) in some ways exemplify this idea.

Many eyewitness reports of UFOs highlight how these objects never follow what we perceive as our predictable rules, or mechanics. UFO's are outlier artifacts that come and go as they wish. Often explained away as "advanced technology." I am not saying I know the answer, but I have to ask. What if it is simply that they, like the game developer, do not need to abide by the mechanics since they control the mechanics?

Surviving Death And Living To Tell About It

NDE's have a similar pattern. The majority of people who have died and come back from clinical death have conveyed similar patterns of experiences. In these experiences time, space and consciousness do not follow the same rules as we know them. It's often a chaotic experience.

People who have experienced NDE's, describe peeling away from their body and hovering over or around the scene. They are able to watch what is going on around their body. At the same time a person experiencing an NDE is able to perceive things happening in a completely different locale, without leaving where they are presently. There is almost always a tunnel or white light that feels loving, comforting and warm. With absolutely no perception of time as we define it.

You Have More Work To Do!

People often describe the same things during the NDE experience. And they often end the same way. Someone tells them, "You have more work to do, it's not your time." Followed by a pulling feeling, ending with them coming back to life.

Yet, somehow they remember these experiences even though they are clinically brain dead. Millions of people have experienced these undeniable and interesting phenomena. Always the person comes back with a completely different view on this existence. What could it be that changes our outlook so quickly and significantly?

Are we all just players in a game called Earth? Each time being reborn, or revived because we still have more lives to play. Are we bound by the physical mechanics defined by another intelligent life form? It is impossible to know of course.

My Personal Brushes With Death

I've had some interesting experiences in my life that are un undefinable. There was one time when I thought I was dying. Which actually turned out to be a gratifying experience for me and shifted my perspective on death. I had blacked out after spending a long time in a very hot, hot spring.

I Thought To Myself, I Am Going To Die Right Here In This Field

We were visiting a beautiful soundless place called Summer Lake, OR. It was so lovely and peaceful. There was a field about 50 yards long that separated our cabin from the baths. I stepped out of the water and walked about 10 feet. Suddenly, feeling woozy, I was no longer able to stand. I fell to my knees, then on all fours, with my hands trembling and the bones in them vibrating. That feeling like when you hit your funny bone. Except in both arms and hands at once. I thought to myself, here it is, I am going to die right here, right now, alone in this field. I am having a heart attack. Then I blacked out.

The feeling after my blackout was somewhat like other people's descriptions of their NDE experiences. I saw the white light, and felt warm and comfortable. But what I found most interesting about myself before I blacked out. I calmly accepted that this was the end, I lived a good life and now it is over. My wife was in the cabin. But as this was happening I thought to myself, I am not going to call out for help.

I don't believe I actually died, rather just blacked out. But at the time I thought I was having a heart attack. It turned out to be a very gratifying experience for me because it gave a sense of comfort in how I would approach my own death. I wasn't afraid, and I didn't panic. Which made me happy.

I don't know how long I was out but then suddenly I came to. Lying in the grass, face down. I was still alive, I muttered to myself, "must be more work to do" and sorta chuckled. Dusted myself off and went back to the cabin and ate lunch.

Another Time In Thailand Was Filled With Laughter

There was another time in Thailand where something similar happened. However, the experience wasn't like at the hot spring where I thought, oh wow I am dying. I had just finished an hour massage, and some acupuncture. The "master", as we referred to the owner of the business, was removing the cups from a bit of cupping he had done on my shoulder and neck to finish out the session. I said, "I think I'm going to black out now" and did. And went to the most amazing, warm, happy white light filled place I have ever been.

I remember it distinctly, I was so incredibly happy, and laughing the entire time. I didn't want to leave and felt very content. For what I'm told was four minutes my wife and the master stood over me trying to revive me. Then slowly I could feel myself resisting this annoying pressure.

The master was firmly pressing two fingers right above my lip, under the center of my nose. There is apparently a pressure point there that can help with people who have had cardiac arrest. It was so annoying that I couldn't resist it and I came to.

They were relieved, but I was actually a bit annoyed when I opened my eyes. My wife said, "you stopped breathing and we thought you died!" I don't know if I actually died. But I will never forget how amazing and happy I felt. I was literally laughing the entire time I was out. And this positive feeling continued for weeks.

My Strong Sense Of Spirits

I have also had several experiences with what can only be referred to as spirits. Which lends credence to the ideas, reported from people who have experienced an NDE, that there are spirits here that we just cannot see. I seem to have a natural sense for this.

For example, when I enter a house or location, right away I will get a certain feeling if it is haunted. Like my wife's friend's apartment in Bangkok's Chinatown. It was in a really old, large building, with many units right on the Chao Phraya river. I didn't like to go over there and told them it was haunted on my first visit. He just laughed and said, "no way" in his French accent.

Our Encounter With The Spirit Of A Child

One night my wife and I were house sitting for them. I was dreading going to sleep because the bedroom was where the spirit's energy was so strong. So I played Playstation until late. After we go to sleep, around 3AM, I am having a dream. In this dream a small girl about 7 or 8 years old was staring at me from a short distance. I felt like she wanted to tell me, or show me something.

What was even more interesting about this experience. In the moments before I started having my dream, my wife was having a dream that there was someone knocking on the bedroom door. She had woken up and gone to the bedroom door, opened it, looked into the living room, closed the door, and got back into bed. Right after she had done this I started dreaming about the person staring at me.

Not long after she had gotten back into the bed I woke up. The first thing I noticed was our cat standing on the foot of the bed, hair raised, tail up, staring towards the bedroom door. So I look over in the direction of the door and there is the figure of a little blonde white girl, with long hair holding a doll, staring back at me. It was just like in the movies! As this is happening my wife noticed that I was sitting up in bed. When she sat up and turned to me and spoke, the little girl ran off through the wall.

Something Happened In The Hallway

On the other side of the wall was the outside hallway that connects the elevator with all the apartments on that floor. It has a strangely low railing and view of the outdoor, inner courtyard below. Somehow, I knew that this little girl died by falling over this railing and she wanted to show me. I had this unsettled feeling that someone pushed her.

After I told my wife what had just happened she informed me about her dream. We couldn't believe how our dreams aligned with the events that had just taken place. There was no way either one of us was going back to sleep. So we agreed to go back to our house and I never went to that apartment again.

When I First Moved To Japan

I had another experience in Japan where once again an apparition came to me in my dream. When I first moved to Tokyo I lived in an area called Numabukuro right next to this nice park with very big trees. A friend of mine, whom I met in New York City, owned the apartment there.

Since she was living in NYC, she let me lease this apartment when I first arrived in Japan. The hairs on my neck and arms are standing up right now as I type this. A very unhappy male spirit occupies this apartment.

My First Encounter With This Dark Spirit

I was literally terrified, even during the day, to go into one of the bedrooms which was being used for storage. I always kept this door closed. At night this spirit would come into the bedroom where I slept and stand over me in bed.

I could feel his cold breath on me, poking me in my sleep. He would torture me by standing over me in my dreams poking me, making me shiver. Every single night without fail I would wake up suddenly feeling like someone was in the room standing over me.

This would go on all night every couple hours I would wake up. It got to the point where I anticipated it and would wake up because I could hear the door creaking open. Even when I closed the door before sleeping. I would wake up and it would be wide open. Even after I closed it and put a shoe against it. When I woke up the door would be open.

Then one day I had sushi for lunch with the mother of my friend. That night I ended up with terrible food poisoning and almost died. It was so bad. I felt like my stomach was going to come out of my mouth after vomiting for two days straight. I ended up at the hospital. I'd never been as sick since.

After about a month of living in this apartment I couldn't take it anymore. I started sleeping in the living room with the lights on, under the kotatsu. Which is a low, wooden table frame covered by a futon, or heavy blanket, upon which a table top sits. Underneath is a heat source and it's super cozy. For some reason it was better to be out of the bedroom. Although, I would wake up sometimes and could feel the spirit watching me from the hall between the bedrooms. I ended up moving as soon as I could find a new place. I will never forget this experience of being tortured by a ghost. I've never experienced anything like that to this day.

Our Energy Is All That Endures

Fortunately, or unfortunately, depending on your point of view, humans don't really live that long in the grand scheme of things. But what about our energetic subconsciousness? There are many documented cases of children remembering their past life in great detail. If energy can never be created or destroyed, then how old are we truly?

Sure in human physical life terms a few hundred years is a long time, but not to the universe. What is our comparison? In what context can humans compare time? Taking this statement with a grain of salt. How do humans even know how old the universe is?

The idea that we can look back into time through shaped glass. Observing light signatures of varying wavelengths to measure time, it's not an easy concept to grasp. How can we know for sure, this is true?

Bang! Now This All Exists

Suddenly, a big bang. An ever expanding universe. Now this all exists. It makes me wonder. When a video game is created, if it too is witness to a big bang. Then suddenly all the game's world exists. Imagine the metaverse. As time goes by, the developer builds, adds architecture and life expanding the footprint.

Oscar Wilde wrote in 1889, "Life imitates Art far more than Art imitates Life." This is known as an anti-mimesis point of view. When compared to Aristotle's mimesis, "art imitates life." From this I pose a question. Is our art, using a video game or the metaverse as an example, imitating our existence? It would seem to be so. And if our existence, our life, is some higher being's art or game. Then our life is imitating art. While our art, or game, is imitating our life. Sounds pretty Rick & Morty to me.

Wilde further states that anti-mimesis, life imitating art, "results not merely from Life's imitative instinct, but from the fact that the self-conscious aim of Life is to find expression, and that Art offers it certain beautiful forms through which it may realise that energy."

85% Of Everything That Exists Is Dark Matter - What That Is, No Human Knows

What exactly is "this" within which we exist? Scientists suppose 85% of the Universe is dark matter. How do they know 85%? What is dark matter? They don't know, but they know it exists, and it makes up the majority of our Universe. I certainly don't know the answer and think these ideas create more questions than answers. Searching for answers is one of the things that keeps us going. Giving us purpose.

Other scientists have even hypothesized that there must be a mirror world right next to ours to account for right spinning neutrinos. Since, for some unknown reason, in our world neutrinos only spin to the left. Maybe our world is the Upside-Down. The upside-down to left spinning neutrinos. Maybe in the left spinning neutrino dimension there is no corruption, everyone gets along, is happy and healthy.

Physicists believe spinning neutrinos are somehow connected to dark matter's function. Even if we have no idea what we are looking for. Like making art, the process is a part of the solution. In this case discovery is the process of creation.

We Are So Very Small

Our concept of time and space is so small. Like a crumb of dust, on a crumb of dust, of the cosmos. Consider the size of the Sun when compared to Earth. Our Sun is more than 100 times the size of Earth and is said to make up 99.8% of all the mass in our solar system. Look out the window of an airplane. Humans are nothing but ants. Tiny little ants.

Our physical world's mass is pretty much meaningless at this scale. Everything humans do. Everything that ever was and will ever be created by human beings began from stardust and shall be returned to stardust and forgotten. All of our buildings, books, monuments, and machines. Every single physical thing, including our bodies will return to our original particle state.

We Are All Made From Stardust

To quote Ali Sundermier again, "About 99 percent of your body is made up of atoms of hydrogen, carbon, nitrogen and oxygen. You also contain much smaller amounts of the other elements that are essential for life. While most of the cells in your body regenerate every seven to 15 years, many of the particles that make up those cells have actually existed for millions of millennia. The hydrogen atoms in you were produced in the big bang, and the carbon, nitrogen and oxygen atoms were made in burning stars. The very heavy elements in you were made in exploding stars." I mean you have to ask. What are we truly? Allegedly, billions of years old if you consider us at a molecular level.

In my opinion. Nothing we do is really significant or important in any way in the grand scale of the physical Universe. Only working on the energy that binds us, our energetic subconsciousness. Finding the right frequency to vibrate with the quantum field that surrounds us. Enabling the unwinding of our DNA back into energy that can never be created, nor destroyed.

Life In A Bubble

Humanity lives in a bubble, quite literally and metaphorically. Yet, we are poisoning this planet like a virus does a cell. Creating waste until the environment has been ruined beyond repair. All in the name of greed, consumption, and reproduction. Is that the reason humans exist? To just endlessly consume, breed and lay waste? Are we a virus and the Earth a cell?

The only meaning derived from living is the one you give to yourself. Many people say they live for their kids. If this was true. Then wouldn't people, who live for their kids, make their best effort to be certain their kids have a better living environment? One that's free of pollution, chemicals, and toxins. How could anyone say they are living for their children, yet not act as custodians of food, of the planet and nature?

Are we all so disconnected from the life force that sustains us? Without the environment of Earth's climate, soil, microbiome and clean water. There is no future for children. Except one of misery and suffering. Life is often said to be "what you make it." This is quite literally and metaphysically true. Right now our actions are making life less and less good for our children.

Owning Our Smallness

Being insignificant in itself is not a motivating thought. Actually owning humanity's insignificance and smallness. Being a nobody is hard to grasp and accept. Those in positions of power always act in a way as to be great, to be somebody in history. Controlled by ego.

Rulers seize lands and say they are doing so to reclaim the "motherlands" or to make their country great, or to liberate people from an oppressor. It's always taken from someone else. Not very often is it given to someone else. Every now and then these gestures are altruistic. In reality, more often than not, they are done for power, greed, or to be remembered historically. However grand these egocentric gestures are presented, the achievements mean nothing in the true scale of time.

Instead The People Suffer

Many times the method to go about these reclamations involves great strife, death, and suffering for everyday people. We need only to look at what is happening in Ukraine for an example. The majority of people just want to live and love in peace.

This negative egocentric or machismo energy does nothing for the collective of humanity. To be great, in my opinion, is to live in peace with all mankind and nature. Which means destroying the Ego.

Countless Hours Of Pointless Toil

The things we take so seriously, like our jobs, possessions, and daily tasks. For the most part, they are just utterly pointless expenditures of energy. "Countless hours of pointless toil," an artist I once knew liked to say. Is that all we are here to do, expend energy and fulfill tasks? We spend so much time doing meaningless errands and consuming.

As you have probably already noticed I enjoy theoretical physics and find quantum theory fascinating. These are truly incredible concepts that scientists are only just beginning to discover. Makes me wonder how long before they are disproven! However, the more I learned, the more it made me realize how utterly pointless everything we do in the physical world is.

Our Energetic Output Matters Most

Since, it is the energetic world that matters most. What we do energetically has the most impact and meaning. When I first started to understand String Theory, for example, it made me somewhat depressed. To think about the measure of time and scale. Yet, it doesn't have to be that way. All I needed to do was change my point of view. I started to think of everything in energetic terms.

I started asking myself. What is it that I am doing each day that creates positive energetic force? Because there is plenty of negative annoyance we each have to put up with every day. It is easy to complain. I seemed to like to complain a lot. Being born in New Jersey and all. Fuhgetaboutit!

So just going about tasks. I began to be conscious in terms of, what is the energy I am sharing. And, whether you realize it or not, negative energy takes a toll on us and others. And it's contagious. For every one negative interaction we have. Energetically it takes about five positive ones to counteract that single negative interaction, according to research done by John Gottman and Robert Levenson.

There Is A Chemical Reason Negativity Sticks With Us

Fear, rejection and criticism cause the release of cortisol in our brain which can shut down our ability to reason and think critically. In a sense this reverts us back to our animal modality, causing us to either "freeze or appease." This can explain some of what I mentioned earlier about groupthink.

We appease, to avoid negative encounters, ones which we cannot be sure if they will bring about conflict. "The self is more motivated to avoid bad self-definitions than to pursue good ones. Bad impressions and bad stereotypes are quicker to form and more resistant to disconfirmation than good ones." – Roy F. Baumeister, Ellen Bratslavsky, Catrin Finkenauer and Kathleen D. Vohs – Review of General Psychology, Bad is Stronger Than Good.

"A single traumatic experience can have long-term effects on the person's health, wellbeing, attitudes, self-esteem, anxiety, and behavior; many such effects have been documented." This means that you are directly responsible for the times you have created negative experiences for other people.

Good Feeling Chemicals Metabolize Faster Than Bad Ones

Positive interactions also stimulate chemical production in the brain. When you get a compliment, for example, the interaction produces oxytocin which is a feel good hormone. However, oxytocin metabolizes quicker than cortisol. This is why bad interactions outweigh good ones and why we tend to have a stronger memory of, or dwell on negative interactions more than positive ones. This is what psychologists refer to as "negative bias". I will talk more about negative bias in chapter six from a different perspective.

When you are going about your day, take into consideration that negativity is contagious and much easier to keep and share. Making it easy to complain, be rude, or be unappreciative and detached. To act entitled.

I personally make a point to do my best to share positivity in my interactions throughout the day. Even if I am grumpy. Regardless of whether negativity is being received. Each person has their own thing and perceptions they are dealing with.

Peace Of Mind Is Love And Compassion

The Dalai Lama says, "The real source of peace of mind is love and compassion; not the love we feel for those who are close to us, but an unlimited sense of altruism, a love that can be extended to all beings, including your enemy, which all human beings are capable of." Imagine if all day you only have negative interactions. We all have probably had these kinds of days and know how it feels. So then we should also recognize these negative feelings linger, sometimes for days.

In a positive feedback loop we all try to minimize our negative impact and maximize our positive impact on other people's lives as much as possible. Building up rather than tearing down. Personally, I feel bad when I negatively impact someone's life. And this can create a negative feedback loop. Which, I believe, in turn creates bad karma. Or in other words a negative feedback loop.

Old Dogs Learning New Tricks

Humans only know what we are told, have learned, and been trained. In many ways we are like really smart dogs. Until we learn or discover some new tricks. We will keep doing as we have been trained. Humanity could be anything, in any paradigm. Humans could live in holes like gophers. Defining certain grasses, or qualities of dirt to be luxurious or delicacies and so forth. And this would be totally normal in this imagined alternate reality. Because we were born into it and everyone else was doing it.

It's possible then, to surmise humanity exists in a need-to-know network. As in, humans in "The Network Earth" just don't need to know. To exist on this planet. Keeping it simple. Like a machine with a set of tasks has no idea about anything besides those tasks. Humans could be serving some function or simulating something on a timeline that just doesn't match with our life scale.

All we have are our limited set of processors. How can a human comprehend that which is beyond its realm of processing or understanding? Is it possible to imagine what a 5th or 6th dimensional being will look like? Will the human eye even be able to witness the sight? Human eyes only see in a very narrow spectrum of light. So many things are just beyond the recognition of a human's limited range of sensors and processorial understanding. Maybe we are built this way on purpose.

Knowing Why We Are Here Would Contaminate The Outcome

Think about it. Maybe if the big picture was known, then humans might stop doing it. Whatever it is we are doing, which seems to be fulfilling tasks. Imagine you knew that this life is totally pointless. Besides how I frame it here, pretend that you had secret knowledge. You know this existence is a simulation. That you are just an avatar. Or that you are a player in a game. Wouldn't this knowledge cause you to change your behavior?

In a way, this goes back to the idea of collapsing the wave function. By observing something, you bring it into existence or change the outcome. By observing the knowledge that this existence is actually a simulation, you might change the outcome, altering the reliability of the simulation. Maybe even crashing the whole system contaminating the outcome. Scientists take many careful precautions, making sure that their data doesn't get corrupted. One would imagine that an experiment at the scale of the Universe might be a costly, time- consuming endeavor.

Moving Forward With Only The Directions Given To Us

I tend to liken humanity to a Mars rover. Testing, sampling, document-ing, excavating and moving forward without any direction (other than that which is given to us). Without any greater truth really.

If human beings, as carbon dating has shown, have existed on Earth for millions of years. Then why do millions of people worship gods from books merely a few thousand years old? Why accept something that can never truly be known? Shouldn't we be skeptical at best? Like all of our knowledge.

Repeating something, someone else said, is kind of like leaving a voicemail. Push a button. The voicemail plays back to you whatever was said before. Nothing more. No matter how many times you listen.

You can't ask any questions. And the story changes as it is shared from one person, to the next. It's also the only story.

The Search For Objectivity

There can be no objectivity with only one perspective of a story. I believe it is important not to be afraid of making your own story. Not in the sense of making up things, rather, making your life, yours. Not just following the path that is set for us. How will you ever be your greatest manifestation of self? If you do not make the effort to reach out and grab it!

Belief in a God can act as a disconnect for our processor, the brain. It helps to rationalize decision making and events in the physical world. And de-rationalize or simplify the thought process. Allowing decision making to be easier. Just to say, "it is God's will," removes thought and ownership. We become subject to, and more importantly victims of, "God's will." Belief is all humanity has. We are always searching for a reason why.

The need to believe there is something greater than us gives reason to live. It is surely more motivating than thinking about the scale of the cosmos. How nothing we do in the physical world has any real significance in relation to time. How in the scope of time spent during our lives is quite possibly pointless.

Serving a purpose greater than we know gives us reason to go on living. Our lifespan is too short to match the scale of the universe. To witness for our own eyes. So we have images, books, and stories. Historical lessons from the past, legends, tales and fables. Passed down and accumulated knowledge (data).

Tales can be a powerful tool for control. Simply the creation of an idea. That there is something beyond our perception. That is keeping track of and watching our actions. Judging us. A being or existence that will punish us or reward us. Taps into a deep psychological force of the unknown. Fear.

CHAPTER SIX

Fear

I believe the fight or flight part of the human brain hasn't caught up with modernity, our environmental stresses and chemical dietary challenges. It used to be simple. Hide from the tiger. Scare monkey away. Eat wild things growing naturally. It's not so simple anymore.

Chemical And Stress Overloaded

Barely one hundred years ago humans didn't have refrigeration. There definitely weren't as many pharmaceuticals, preservatives, and chemical additives in food, water and the air like today. In our current era everyday we are overloaded with toxins, chemicals, advertisements, and information.

Too much is happening at once, attacking our senses, causing stress. We are over-saturated, divided and overloaded. Those in positions of power take advantage of this situation. While making sure to keep things the same.

A key factor to mitigating stress response and keeping healthy is maintaining a healthy diet. Of course I don't consider this a new idea. However, some may not take diet and lifestyle into consideration at all. To be clear: proper diet, mindfulness, meditating, exercising, and maintaining proper gut bacteria balance, limiting toxins, stimulants and depressants—these steps are vital to proper health and control of fear response. Not to mention to live a healthy and happy life in the Anthropocene.

Probiotics And The Gut Brain Connection

There have been some interesting studies done with mice and the probiotic bacteria, lactobacillus. In one such study at McMaster University in Canada. Mice were placed in a stressful situation to measure anxiety and stress response. One at a time a single mouse was placed in a bucket of water. With no way to escape. The goal of this study was to see how gut bacteria might influence brain behavior and stress response.

The control group were just normal mice. Eating normal mice food. The study group had been fed lactobacillus rhamnosus, a probiotic bacteria. The control group, when placed in the water, swam frantically, trying to escape until they were exhausted. The study group—the one fed lactobacillus rhamnosus—swam in a less frantic, thoughtful manner.

After the mice had given up and stopped swimming. The researchers removed them from the water and tested for corticosterone. Corticosterone is the mice version of the human stress hormone, cortisone. They found that the study group, the mice fed lactobacillus rhamnosus, had significantly lower levels of corticosterone than the control group.

The Vagus Nerve

For the second part of the study the scientists severed the vagus nerve. The vagus nerve is the longest nerve in the human body. It contains both motor and sensory functions and runs from the medulla oblongata all the way to the gut. For our purposes here you just need to understand that it connects the stomach to the brain. In man and mice.

When the scientists ran the same tests after severing the vagus nerve. They found that the lactobacillus rhamnosus had absolutely no effect on anxiety reaction or corticosterone production.

This finding suggests that the gut brain connection has an important linkage—more importantly, that there is a link between bacteria in the stomach and chemical function in the brain. Lactobacillus rhamnosus was shown to minimize the production of the fear-inducing hormone corticosterone. This in turn, helped to minimize stress and fear reaction. Enabling clear headed decision making.

Stress And IBS

Another study worth mentioning was done by Jay Pasricha, M.D., Director of Johns Hopkins Center for Neurogastroenterology. In terms of constipation, diarrhea, and Irritable Bowel Syndrome (IBS), researchers are finding that irritation in the gut ends up sending signals to the brain that trigger mood changes. "For decades, researchers and doctors thought that anxiety and depression contributed to these problems. But our studies and others show that it may also be the other way around," Pasricha says. "That's important, because up to 30 to 40 percent of the population has functional bowel problems at some point."

What doctor Pasricha is saying. Stress, anxiety and depression are caused by bowel problems, rather than contributing to the onset of these problems. Scientists have just located the tip of the iceberg when it comes to the gut-brain connection. There are many studies out there showing how gut bacteria affect mood, thinking clarity, and so on.

If you want to learn more. Here are a couple books you should check out; Giulia Enders, Gut: The Inside Story of Our Body's Most Underrated Organ and The Mind-Gut Connection by Emeran Mayer, MD. If you are interested in learning more about your body and how it works. This knowledge will empower and motivate you to eat healthier. It will also improve your quality of life.

Making Your Own Probiotic Rich Foods

Making your own fermented foods at home is a fun hobby. In one sitting you can make months worth of probiotic snacks that contain lactobacillus. If you need help to get started. There's an excellent book by Sandor

Katz called the Art of Fermentation. This book has all the information and recipes you will ever need to ferment almost anything at home.

Something else to keep in mind. There really shouldn't be more than a gram or two of sugar in any type of probiotic food. Ideally, all of the sugar will be fermented out. So with store bought items check the added sugar content. And it's not just sucrose. Sweeteners have 56 different names, which I will detail more later on.

Probiotic foods like sauerkraut, tempeh, miso and pickles shouldn't have any sugar at all. Check the label if you are buying kimchi. Store bought kimchi will often have sugar in it. I make kimchi at home all the time and you can leave out the sugar when you do it yourself. It is not a necessary ingredient.

One other thing to keep in mind. Products listing microflora count on the packaging. If it's counted, there is a very good chance it's added. These are not living, natural probiotics. Many of these products have been heat pasteurized. Which means you are consuming the dead bacteria. The producers then add probiotics back in.

All Gut Health Studies Say The Same Thing

All of the gut related studies out there suggest the same thing: improper microbial gut balance, affects decision making, mood, skin health, energy levels and creates a tendency to overreact to stress and fear. Bad bacteria will make you unhealthy and can cause you to make poor decisions.

When you pair these facts with some other fascinating psychologically based brain studies the picture becomes even clearer.

The Political Brain

Empirical evidence suggests that political identification is less about how humans are opinionated or view the world. Instead it turns out that the brains of conservatives and liberals are actually physically different.

Scientists at University College London found that those "who identify themselves as conservatives have a larger amygdala than self-described liberals." The amygdala is the fear processing center of the human brain. This finding suggests that conservatives are more prone to react stronger to perceived threats.

In another study published in 2008 in the National Health Institute, National Library of Medicine. Researchers found that liberal minded students tend to seek adventure and travel more. Whereas, conservative minded students tend to live a more orderly lifestyle and enjoy familiarity.

"Although political views have been thought to arise largely from individuals' experiences, recent research suggests that they may have a biological basis. We present evidence that variations in political attitudes correlate with physiological traits. In a group of 46 adult participants with strong political beliefs, individuals with measurably lower physical sensitivities to sudden noises and threatening visual images were more likely to support foreign aid, liberal immigration policies, pacifism, and gun control, whereas individuals displaying measurably higher physiological reactions to those same stimuli were more likely to favor defense spending, capital punishment, patriotism, and the Iraq War. Thus, the degree to which individuals are physiologically responsive to threat appears to indicate the degree to which they advocate policies that protect the existing social structure from both external (outgroup) and internal (norm-violator) threats."

Negativity Bias

In a 2012 study published in The Royal Society, conservatives were shown to have "negativity bias." A bit like I mentioned earlier, when negativity is contagious. In this study researchers monitored subjects' eye movements. When shown two images—one "positive," like a cute kitten, and one "negative," like a car wreck—liberal identifying participants would look at the cute kitten first. Conservatives, on the other hand, would look at the car wreck first.

Psychologists refer to this as "negativity bias." Meaning conservatives' attention is skewed toward threats. Making the world a scarier place for conservatives. University of Central Arkansas social psychologist Paul Nail says, "Conservatism, apparently, helps to protect people against some of the natural difficulties of living. The fact is we don't live in a completely safe world. Things can and do go wrong. But if I can impose this order on it by my worldview, I can keep my anxiety to a manageable level." In this situation for the conservative mindset it's all about managing anxiety. That may be a reason so many gun owners identify as conservatives. Guns, of course, make people feel safe.

Feeling Safe Versus Feeling Threatened

From the Scientific American, Unconscious Reactions Separate Liberals and Conservatives, September 2012: "When people feel safe and secure, they become more liberal; when they feel threatened, they become more conservative. Research conducted by Paul Nail and his colleague in the weeks after September 11, 2001, showed that people of all political persuasions became more conservative in the wake of the terrorist attacks. Meanwhile, in an upcoming study, a team led by Yale University psychologist Jaime Napier found that asking Republicans to imagine that they possessed superpowers and were impermeable to injury made them more liberal."

This is a really important piece of information here. Take some time to consider the meaning of this quote. Boiled down it means - more terrorism, more wars and more chaos, will in turn make people generally become more conservative. If you want to push a society to be more restrictive, and increase your power structures what do you do? Create a climate of fear and sow chaos of course.

What happened after 911? Everything got tighter, more laws, more powers for government and less for citizens. I was living in the East Village when 911 happened. I watched it all unfold and even went down there to take photos. The felling of those towers defied laws of physics and structural engineering.

Politicians Use Fear And Anxiety To Decrease Freedoms

Politicians are well aware of this type of research because they studied political science at Ivy League schools and became experts in being politicians. As a politician your job is to manipulate people to side with you. If you are a politician, pushing a conservative agenda. Trying to crack down on civil liberties, or increase your power. It is in your interest to scare people. To create misinformation, conspiracy, drama and even perform false (black) flag operations. This is no conspiracy theory either, this is in practice right now, and has been happening for as long as there have been top down societies.

These studies I mention suggest that the sort of information, physical events and the perspective from which the human brain processes it, triggers predictable, known outcomes. In conservatives with their larger, or more developed, amygdala, it is easier for the process to bypass the critical thinking part of the brain and connect directly to the hardwired fight or flight part.

Fear And Control Never Equals Freedom

Knowing this information we should then consider that media consumption and dietary preferences are two more parts of the reaction machine. Why are conservative news and conservative politicians always talking about the crime rate and freedom? Putting out media that thrives on outrage and pushing an agenda towards less freedoms, but selling it as freedom. It's upside-down manipulation and programming.

Observe how the fear based media complexes exist in America. It should come as no surprise that experts in the field of conservative media, know about these psychological studies, and are pushing a steady diet of fear, anxiety inducing, reactionary news stories. Complete with the imagery to catch your attention. With culture war chants against things like the "War on Christmas" which supposedly rejects Christian values. Or the "War on Meat" which rejects ideas of a healthy diet and lifestyle. In favor of the freedom to hurt your own health while ignoring the massive detriment to the environment meat production creates. Portraying eating meat as masculine.

This is all so blatantly control based messaging meant to keep the consumerist status quo and support existing entrenched financial architectures. You will understand more in the following chapters. It's all about money, control and power of course. Kinda boring really, to live an entire life searching for just the extensions of those things.

The Portrayal - Masculine Vs. Feminine

How about the constant portrayal of alternative energy as weak and in a negative light? Because it's passive? Why is oil manly? Because macho men dig it from the Earth with big machines and get dirty? Because it makes fire and go-boom!? Wind and solar are passive, so they are feminine?

It's not new information that this programming is all about profits. Conservative media and politicians are selling top down, male dominance, religion and consumption through fear. In doing this they are suggesting people should reject things that will be better for humanity, the planet and themselves. It's better to keep things the way they are. Don't rock the boat, son.

This is how the media and politicians prop up the status quo while pretending the opposite. They send out these triggering messages accompanied by reactionary imagery. Riling people up, getting them to react without thinking. Since, the conservative mindset with their larger amygdala are easily riled up. They take the bait. The media and politicians manipulate anyone who is fearful or anxious easily. And it's so much bigger than just this.

Meanwhile, the same people putting out misinformation say that they are just being free thinkers, asking questions. Stirring the pot and turning up the heat lets humans' own brains simmer, and do their dirty work for them. When you can't control the voices in your head it's easy to mistake what is reality.

The Fear Of Something New - The Fear Of Loss

It is always "they", some invisible outsiders, who are going to take something away from you. "They " are going to change the things that are so familiar to you. "They" want to replace you. The way this information is presented to us is meant to divide and create fear. Meant to elicit an anxiety induced, reactionary, hardwired reflex. Opposition to the other, or the outsider is our caveman instinct.

The definition of the word "conserve" from Merriam Webster: "*to avoid wasteful or destructive use of*" or "*to keep in a safe or sound state.*" Conservative political principles are just that. Reserving the past ways. Keeping safe in the conservative perspective of order and familiarity. Fearing the unknown, the outsider, and rejecting the new.

This is exactly why conservative media is always talking about freedom, crime, immigration and safety. But how is it freedom? Actually, the definition of conservative is the opposite. Freedom is not equal to restriction.

This messaging is tapping into anxiety. By constantly saying we have to conserve the traditional or familiar ways of thinking and doing. Putting conservative minds on alert, always giving them something to defend against. An outsider, a threat, the loss of something familiar. It's clear as day in the messaging if you start to pay attention. Causing the conservative mind to want to control the disorder, to take action. I ask a serious question here. Isn't the definition of control the opposite of freedom?

The Best Way To Keep Things The Same

The goal is of course to keep reinforcing the status quo. Therefore, by keeping the conservative reaction machine and anxiety ramped up to maximum. Nothing will change or things will become more conservative, and even more restrictive. Looking at this objectively, these ideas seem hypocritical. If a person says "don't tread on me," give me freedom to do what I want. While at the same time is treading on other people and taking away their freedoms. This in the end, turns out to be less freedom for everyone.

A Morning Consult poll found, "26% of the U.S. population qualified as highly right-wing authoritarian." It begs the question. Can you name one place in the world with an authoritarian government that has more freedoms than a democratic one? I think the ideas are mutually exclusive.

The conservative mind keeps following a familiar black and white perspective. Authoritarianism is at once less thoughtful and easy for those craving order in their lives. Activating familiar subconscious brain patterns. Firing solidly wired neural pathways. Keeping close to what is known. Out of fear, need to control and anxiety arise. Yet, control will never be freedom. Which, when you think about it, is perfect logic if you live in the upside-down.

Fear Is Money And Power

The media and politicians are regularly triggering humans, absolutely doing it purposefully. Because it makes them a lot of money. This sort of information and presentation interrupts the connection to rational thought. And that interruption makes it much easier to rile people up and get them to take action without thinking. A population that just does and doesn't think about what it is they are doing is just a flock of sheep. Again there is no freedom here.

Unfortunately, it is very difficult to change this type of mindset. I personally believe there is a big part of this that has to do with diet and lifestyle choices. It would seem conservative leaning humans reject anything that doesn't fit within their limited worldview. Including ideas that conflict with what is already pre-conditioned thought patterns and behaviors, hardwired into the brain. These humans skip over the logical and rational decision making part of the brain. Rejecting objectivity, facts or any knowledge that conflicts or confronts their own world view.

A System Based On Rejection

Regardless of new knowledge, systems availability, or ideas, the conservative mindset rejects things that challenge what they believe. The pathways are so neurologically hardwired. It will take a lot of dedicated work on a conservative person's part to accept new information and ideas to change these thought patterns.

This process becomes even more difficult if their peers are constantly challenging them and rejecting their process of change. There is no interest in dedication to learning new ways of thinking, acting, being or importantly, challenging personal beliefs. Going outside of the comfort zone. And so the sole purpose becomes resisting the outsider, acting with negativity bias. How could these individuals ever give themselves the opportunity to make meaningful positive change in their lives?

Evolution Means Changing

One way to evolve is to change diet, habits, environment and thinking processes. Imagine how many ways life on Earth has had to adapt over millions of years. It has to be purposeful and done with dedication and it means life or death. Learning to be open minded and adopting new behaviors is a choice. Choosing to take these actions will wire new neural pathways. Disengaging the old neural pathways that are not being used.

There are many studies which show how fear and anxiety rule the conservative mindset. This mindset feels safety in numbers and like-mindedness. This is precisely why if one of the group attempts to change, they are bullied back into submission. This is cult-like behavior or even worse, authoritarianism. None of which equals "freedom."

It's Like Recovering From Drug Addiction

In some ways this is no different than heroin addiction. When an addict gets clean, they can never go back to their old circle of friends or environment. The same is true here. By returning to their old environs the conservative mindset would potentially habituate back into the same familiar ideas and paradigm. When you look at the psychology of this, it's almost an impossible task for the most conservative to evolve.

Drawing on the information I've just provided. Imagine an individual with a conservative mindset having to give up all of what is familiar to them, including their friends. Solely so they can evolve and learn to think and act in a new way. Considering that the majority of conservative humans live in rural areas, don't like to travel and crave familiarity. Changing thinking for this type of mindset would be a monumental undertaking. Rejecting everything that they once stood for.

Not Changing With The World Creates Feelings Of Resentment

Often these same humans state they feel left behind. They feel resentful because the world is changing around them. They want to fight it! Here is another really important dot. From a psychological viewpoint, humans are more likely to fight for something they are losing than to fight for something to gain.

Yet, these individuals are being left behind, precisely because they refuse to change. This feeling is therefore of their very own choosing and doing, a creation of their own self. Negativity bias strikes again. To manage their anxiety they must subjugate everyone else. Control is the only way. In the conservative worldview society is not allowed to progress. We must instead stay the same or even worse, go backward.

Victimhood Never Claims Ownership

Claiming victimhood many will actively resist these types of statements, taking no ownership of thoughts and actions based out of fear. Because these behaviors are built from fight or flight. It is a black and white decision. There is no rationalization of these types of decisions.

Unfortunately, these very humans will become, and are, a barrier to the future paradigm, holding humanity's evolution back. If you look around at the present state of politics in America, you can see this is on clear display. We must change as a whole. Yet instead we are like a cell dividing into two different organisms.

The Liberal Mindset

A liberal mindset, generally speaking, tends to register on the more flexible and accepting end of the spectrum. This mindset is more inclusive and open. Going with the flow. Less concerned with defense and more with offense.

Liberal minded humans did not react so strongly to the violent imagery and sounds mentioned in the previous studies. The liberal mind with its smaller amygdala is more accepting of new paradigms, interested in discovery, new ideas, new experiences and thought patterns. "Liberal" defined by Merriam Webster: *"one who is open-minded or not strict in the observance of orthodox, traditional, or established forms or ways."*

Not to say that there's no liberal fear based media. It swings both ways of course. But maybe it is slightly less effective considering the circumstances. More importantly, there are many grey areas in the middle. It's possible to hold both conservative and liberal beliefs at the same time.

I use the political argument in this chapter to illustrate the bigger picture, which is how much power and control fear has over us. How it is used and how different types of people are more sensitive to it. And if you are conservative this knowledge could very much help you to gain objectivity. Because, above all, you have to know yourself the most, first. Before you can start to break down the "why's" of what you do.

Descriptive And Opposite

Seems like liberal and conservative definitions are pretty literal in their description. When relating to human political traits in America, it would seem that the conservatives hate the liberals. Each is the other's antagonist. Conservatism seems to operate strictly to do. What they like to refer to as "owning the libs" or "triggering the libs." This is a control tactic. Controlling others through intimidation. Hence the terminology, "owning" and "triggering."

Yet, what we don't see nearly as often. Liberal minded people take this same sort of approach. Sure liberals will "troll" conservatives. In my opinion this is mostly due to the hypocrisy. I believe the liberal mindset does not make decisions strictly based on controlling or poking fun of conservative individuals. I'm sure there's a lot more to it than my very basic, generalized simplifications. Even though the title has the word political in it. This book is not really meant to be political. And this is a hard chapter to write from my perspective. But it's an important point to distinguish how the brains of two ends of political theory can actually react differently to information.

Darwinian Theory

A study published in the Journal of Health Psychology explored the jock versus nerd stereotypes. Interestingly enough, it appears that jocks tend to find more enjoyment in physical activity. Whereas nerds tend to find more enjoyment in what the researchers called "need for cognition," or thinking.

Which brings an interesting thought to mind. Following Darwinian theory, survival of the fittest. In order to succeed, reproduce, and survive, physical strength and anxiety were the requirements. Imagine two deer smashing antlers. The bigger and stronger deer gets to spread his DNA. This deer also grows bigger and lives longer because he is very much risk averse. Other studies suggested that nerds tend to be lower in reproduction rates than jocks, lending credence to the Darwinian method.

Using myself as an example. The more I exercise the more likely I am to talk to a woman and want to have sex. Strenuous exercise raises testosterone levels. Whereas thinking does not. So this all could be a part of it. However, in the Anthropocene this seems like it could be reversing.

Revenge Of The Nerds

Thinking is becoming a more dominant trait. And maybe thinking isn't exactly the correct word to use here. But let's go with it. Look at our business leaders. They are all nerds! The most valuable companies in America have all been founded by thinkers. Some of those nerds are also conservative.

I often wonder if being very wealthy makes people more conservative. Since conservative political priorities often favor the wealthy by cutting taxes, busting unions and reducing regulation. Maybe it is solely self serving. Just a thought.

This brings me to another example. Since the polling used political affiliation, I will use their terminology in this example. Polling had revealed that in the 2016 and 2018 elections, in general, people voting Republican tended to be less educated and without a college degree. Whereas Democratic voters tended to be more educated and have more advanced degrees as well. However, 25 years ago this statistic was completely reversed.

Change Is Inevitable, But Not Before We Hit Rock Bottom

The world is changing and conservatives are being left behind. In this instance simply because of a lack of education, or "need for cognition." Granted there are many very well educated conservative people. They are however, not the majority. Conservative politicians these days also seem to say the darndest things.

Take Senator Ted Cruz for example. And there are many other fine examples. Ted Cruz is just an easy target. He went to Princeton and Harvard, both Ivy League schools. Yet, some of the statements these politicians make, make absolutely no sense at all. With so much education you have to wonder, why is that? Creating culture war arguments simply to rile up their base and keep them engaged. This is a race to the bottom.

Jocks Versus Nerds

Again, loosely generalizing here, there are exceptions. (I can't wait to hear what the critics say.) One might infer that liberals in the 21st century tend to be nerds. While conservatives tend to be jocks. I know this statement may sound controversial, but bear with me. Obviously, there are caveats in this train of thought, but I want to put this in the perspective of what I have already mentioned.

Conservatives want to keep the world the way it is. The tough guy always wins. Men are manly! We tan our testicles! (This one's for you Tucker) Imagine the jocks in high school always bullying the nerds around. The jocks were the popular kids. They got the girls. For as long as humanity has existed we have lived in the jocks dominion, where the strong rule.

Maybe with technology. Our current society is shifting. The strong archetype is becoming less valuable whereas thinking is finding more value. It's not uncommon to hear reports that robots will replace humans doing many manual labor jobs. And they already are.

Our Changing Society Is Just Beginning

This could be where all the right wing rage against "Wokeism" comes in. We are becoming a society that is built less on hard work done with physical grit. To one that is more inclusive of women and LGBTQ people. One where it's less that the masculine man always dominates and the woman stays home with the kids to cook. A world where it is now work hard from home with your brain. A society of feelings, ease and convenience.

I'm not saying that all the manual labor jobs have gone away. But a significant portion of the economy has shifted away from industrialism. And the real shift hasn't even happened yet. The internet, Google, Microsoft and Apple are barely 40 years old in the sense of popular adoption. Social media and modern tech are barely 30 years old. Our society is changing faster than ever. This type of shift requires learning new skills, changing thinking patterns and adapting. Precisely, what the conservative mindset seems to stand against. Hence all the rage!

Darwin's Last Stand

If you are an American or have been in America anytime in the last couple decades, the political rhetoric and iconography is clear as day. The January 6th insurrection. The talk of civil war, of a race war. The coarseness of our political bodies. Following Darwinian (or Trumpian) logic, the tough and strong should always be the victor. What if society as a whole is moving beyond that?

If we look strictly from an astrological perspective, the Earth's position in the universe is moving out of Pisces and into the age of Aquarius. In Astrology the universe is divided into 12 parts, or constellations. Each is said to express a different part of the human personality.

As the Earth wobbles it takes roughly 2150 years to move through each constellation or sign. Earth moved into Pisces right around the time that Christianity came into being. This is why Christ is often represented as a fish. According to Wikipedia, "the twelve apostles were called the "fishers of men," early Christians called themselves "little fishes," and a code word for Jesus was the Greek word for fish, "Ikhthus.""

Aquarius Is A Water Sign, Feminine And Flexible

Here is what I find interesting about Aquarius and how it aligns with my train of thought. Pisces is the 12th sign in the Zodiac. Since the Zodiac moves counterclockwise, the beginning of Pisces could be said to have marked the end of the last cycle of about 25,920 years. Aquarius is the 11th sign and known as the water bearer.

Water symbolizes flexibility and is a feminine representation. Aquarius is said to be associated with social justice, society, humanitarianism, intelligence, discovery, technology, democracy, freedom, idealism, science and all things futuristic. It's possible to consider these traits as a whole would not seem to be conservative by definition.

Some theorists believe that the age of Aquarius will bring an end to the dominant themes of the last century; racism, sexism, religious intolerance and nationalism, which are said to be traits of Pisces. This all seems to fit with what is happening right now with the human collective subconsciousness. The move from a strength dominated existence into an existence where strength and grit as traits are no longer as necessary as they once were.

The Mother Is The Opposite Of The Father

When you think of a mother, or woman, and the qualities that a mother exemplifies, they are the exact opposite of the father, or man. If we consider the last era, Pisces, was the era of the father. Which happens to also be coded language for God. Like a pendulum swings. Everything starts to make sense.

If you search on the internet "Socialism polls," what pops up first is all the far right websites talking about how Democrats have positive views of Socialism. More view Socialism favorably than Capitalism. Almost half of Generation Z view Socialism favorably.

These media outlets depict this in a negative light because this is exactly what conservative humans have been trained to stand against. Even though all humans will benefit from having a more equitable world, conservatives and liberals alike. Many conservatives will still fight against it. Because as I previously mentioned, humans are more prone to fight for something they are losing than to fight for something to gain.

Each generation wants to move forward. Sometimes the generation before tries to hold progress back. Only now, in my opinion, we are evolving faster than ever. I think it's possible the Earth's position in the universe is moving us into the age of more caring and kindness. Or maybe it is just what is happening regardless of the universe. Maybe this is just solely my opinion. No matter what it is, you can't deny the reality of what is happening around us.

Change Is Inevitable

Either way, we are able to look around and observe this split happening. There are many examples. I believe we are entering an age of the feminine where compassion, thinking and caring is coming into trend. While masculine toughness is going out of trend. Thought and discovery are replacing brute force. The humans who cling to the old way will very obviously be left behind. Evolution is inevitable.

Charles Darwin Also said, "It is not the strongest of the species that survives, nor the most intelligent that survives. It is the one that is the most adaptable to change, that lives within the means available and works co-operatively against common threats."

It is possible, however, that those clinging to the past ways of being may ruin it for everyone. The bully only cares about winning. The costs are never taken into consideration. A man doesn't have or show his feelings. There are humans actively attempting to impede evolution right now and it seems as if they will do anything to retain control. To turn back the clock.

I hope this does not include destroying it for everyone. You could say this is the Yin and Yang of society. A clear example of a physical paradigm that has been created for us right in front of our faces. Used to separate us into tribes. Keeping us fighting against our own best interests and against the "other."

Keeping The Anxiety Cranked Up To Ten

The gut is political in my mind because an imbalanced gut helps to keep the anxiety cranked up. Toxic food creates toxic humans. Our diets and lifestyle choices do somewhat inform our political preferences. As does peer pressure to stick to these diets. Because diets affect our thought processes, behaviors and mood. They are absolutely informing our stress response and much more.

Much of this returns back to our susceptibility to peer pressure and advertising, to cultural norms and how we were raised. How our brains are wired to react since our youth. We possess built in biases and bacteria from our families, diets, and experiences. Many parents, though not all, do not wish their children to think differently than they do. So these tribal structures are re-enforced throughout childhood into adulthood.

My Conservative Father Was Pretty Stereotypical

My father was conservative. He loved football, baseball, playing guitar and being American. I played sports growing up. I always had to be the star player. "Be the best!" he always said. My father coached our football and baseball teams.

In high school I decided to break away from this and started skateboarding. I wanted to explore creativity. This was a time when skateboarding was new and not popular at all. He rejected me and our relationship was never the same. Not until we were much older were we able to reconnect. It was very much about control and being tough with him.

Masculinity Is Bad For Your Health

Masculinity studies have actually shown masculinity to be toxic for our health, planet, and society. Not in the tough guy sense—although if you view it through a political lens, then yes in the tough guy sense as well. These studies were more focused on the idea of having to be a tough guy to keep up with appearances. To keep up with the paradigm.

Somewhere we were made to believe that acting and being certain ways are what it means to be masculine. It's reinforced everyday on TV, in the media and by our leaders. Projecting strength, always fighting, at war with everything. Everything is a crisis to beat up or a war to protect against. Just look at the terminology being used. "War on Christmas," "War on Drugs," "War on Meat," etcetera. Mother Teresa said "I will never attend an anti-war rally; if you have a peace rally, invite me." It's all about the terminology and messaging.

Masculinity As A Political Tool

Masculinity is also a very powerful political cudgel. As shown when we look at the authoritarians and autocrats (and wannabe authoritarians and autocrats) of our time. Masculinity is a great excuse for malfeasance and poor behavior. Never mind the law. He's a man. A man does what he wants, takes what he wants, it's just locker room talk. He wins at all costs!

Masculinity and religion are the tools of dictators and politicians the world over because they operate using fear based, top down, patriarchal ideology. Humans are readily manipulated and distracted with easily activated fear mechanisms and generally opposed to conflict. We become numb to the rhetoric. But the energy doesn't ever become numb. The energy persists and grows.

Imagine The Many Ways Humans Have Existed On This Planet

If you will imagine historically, all the ways we have existed from one generation to the next. From caves and hunter gathers, to farmers, to work-at-home-ers. Our paradigm could be whatever we decide to say it is. Instead, we let those in power set the boundaries for what is acceptable and what is not. When you really think about it we actually don't have free will.

Just like Jack Dorsey said. Human beings are being programmed and have been programmed throughout history. All the way into this very moment. More than ever in this moment, with so much media and advertising saturation. This manipulation has become every minute of every day.

Manipulation Through Media And Conspiracy

Not just through politics and food, but also social media, TV, podcasts, and society as a whole. Would you believe that fake news and negative news stories are six times more likely to be shared on social media (and believed) than true or positive ones? It's unbelievable but true.

The crazier, the more sensational, the more people want to believe it's it. People are losing their minds and the energetic consequences are all too real. The ones pushing these narratives are manifesting their preferred reality. One that is ruled by fear and chaos. Where those in power have lots of control. The strategy of divide and conquer is as old as the famous military tactician, Sun Tzu.

Humans Are Marionettes

Humans have been shaped and molded over millennia by emperors, monarchs, religions, tribal and political parties. Most recently, we are being shaped by corporations, marketing, TV, advertising, and social media. Mostly, this paradigm is benefiting the few. Keeping profits at the top and people at the bottom.

Advertisers and our rulers set the boundaries, make the laws, and pull our strings. Whether conservative or liberal, every single day we must wake up and see that the proverbial "They" have the data and information to micromanage us down to the most minute bacterial levels. And they do it. It's not a conspiracy. This is a fact. Look around and see for yourselves.

Social Media Easily Influences Marionettes

In 2010 Facebook did some internal studies measuring how they were able to swing votes. From an article in Slate, One Facebook Banner Ad Caused 60,000 More People to Vote in the 2010 Elections, September, 2012: "On the day of the 2010 Congressional elections, Facebook ran an experiment on behalf of a research team based at the University of California San Diego. At the top of 61 million users' news feeds, it placed a banner ad that said "Today is Election Day," linked to information about polling places, and showed pictures of the user's Facebook friends who had already clicked an "I Voted" widget on the site. For another

600,000 users, it placed the same informational message, but without the information about the user's friends who had voted. And a control group of 600,000 users got no message at all."

When some elections are decided by only a few hundred or several thousand votes. "It turns out that a single banner message on Facebook directly spurred 60,000 more people to vote in the 2010 election than would have voted otherwise. And research on social contagion effects suggests that another 280,000 people were indirectly influenced to vote by the message."

Imagine a scenario where the CEO of Facebook has a preferred presidential candidate. Facebook could very easily swing an election and they have already done it. I won't delve into all the elections Facebook has already rigged with Cambridge Analytica. You should find out for yourself. There is a great documentary out there called "The Great Hack."

The Power Of The Few Is Too Great And Growing

Just look at a person like Elon Musk for example. Corporations, politicians, billionaires and opinionated media personalities wield way too much power through fear, misinformation, social media, the press and groupthink. Simply because humans are not thinking for themselves.

How many times have you or someone you know just repeated some talking points they saw on TV verbatim? Yet, can't actually back up these positions with facts or evidence? Because chances are high that none exists. We have to come back to reality. Use our objective brain.

In my case I hear it too often in everyday conversations. Fear sells. Fear makes a lot of money! Media as powered by one person or a limited few people could mean the end of a civilized, truly democratic society. Precisely because people are not even bothering to check for facts before sharing, and are 6x more likely to believe the fantastical instead. If the fantastical makes 6x more money than the truth and profits are the only motivation. Do I need to explain further?

Humanity has to get clearheaded, find our focus, detox the body and mind, and come together. We must be strong and learn to stop the knee-jerk reactions. Focusing on building ourselves and everyone else up, instead solely existing to tear others down. Controlling fear is power. To control fear you have to control yourself, your focus and your diet first. But if you can control fear, you awaken a superpower you didn't know you had.

CHAPTER SEVEN

Manipulation

If bacteria in our gut can alter our brain functions, mood, and thinking clarity, then I think it safe to say that consuming a commercial product—made using bacteriological production methods—could have an adverse effect on our health, mental clarity, and even the expression of our genes.

Corn Syrup And Its Derivatives

In this case I am specifically referring to corn syrup and its derivatives, dextrose, maltose and high fructose corn syrup. Highly fermentable sugars made from corn starch. They may seem pretty harmless on the surface since they are made from corn. But, maybe they are not so harmless after all. The majority are made from GMO (genetically modified) corn. When you dig deeper into the production methods and learn more about the process, things become less simple and potentially a lot more harmful to your wellbeing.

The Chemical Process Of Making Corn Syrup

As someone who loves fermentation I was interested to find out as much as I could about the process. First, the starch has to be separated from the corn kernels. They do this by mixing water with sulfur dioxide. Sulfur dioxide is a toxic gas emitted from volcanoes. When you burn a match, that smell is sulfur dioxide gas.

After a few more processes all of the starch has been separated. The producer then uses enzymes excreted from bacteria and fungi. These bacteria and fungi also have been genetically modified to meet commercial production needs for replicability. One of the more common forms of bacterium used is Bacillus licheniformis which is most commonly found in dirt.

Corn Syrup Is Made From Bacterial Excretions

Bacillus species produce enzymes called α-amylase through excretion. Excretion is a nice sounding word but let's put it in context. What is human excrement? Feces, shit, poop, doo-doo whatever you want to call it. It's a waste product in this form and contains genes and DNA. Remember the mice who were given human feces in chapter 4? And those awesome sounding diet pills for human consumption?

The enzyme α-amylase is prevalent in the human body, and is most commonly found in human saliva. What actually is saliva? I'm glad you asked. Saliva is made from your blood. We have glands that filter the water from the blood to make saliva, and tears. This α-amylase enzyme in saliva breaks down starch into maltose and dextrin, which is harmless enough in human form, bearing human based DNA strands.

The fungi used to make corn syrup and its derivatives is Aspergillus. Aspergillus excretes γ-amylase which further helps to convert the oligosaccharides created from the α-amylase into glucose. Like Bacillus, Aspergillus has many different species. Some species are used to make Sake (Japanese rice wine), others are used in medicine. Yet, other forms will make a human sick. Think black mold.

DNA Soup

Here is where it gets interesting. In saliva, depending on your diet, you could have different DNA copies of α-amylase genes. Remember in chapter 4 when I mentioned how the number of DNA/genes and microbiota living in/on the human body significantly outnumber human DNA/genes. Imagine a big old pot of soup. That is what's going on in the human gut and mouth. Human genes, genes from food, fungi genes, bacteria genes, archaea genes all blending together. Food producing corporations are aware of this.

One such brand is Nestlé. Nestlé's former CEO, when asked, is on record referring to water as a human right being an "extreme" argument. I point this out to give a tiny peek into the rationalization of a multi-billion dollar corporation. Of course Nestlé is one of the largest sellers of bottled water on the planet. This kind of thinking should make you start thinking.

Epigenetics, A Little Know Way To Alter Your Genes

I bring up Nestlé because they have hundreds of scientists working on the science and technology of their products. Nestlé, of course, isn't the only company that operates this way. They just happen to be one of the biggest. One field specifically Nestlé focuses on is the epigenetic impacts of diet and lifestyle on individual health. They are proud of this and advertise it. So Nestlé is very well aware of the ability of food to switch genes on and off.

The term epigenetics describes the study of how different biological and environmental signals affect gene expression. There are basically two types of gene expression. The ones you are born with, like your skin tone, and the color of your hair and eyes. Which you can't change, naturally at least. And then there are environmental or epigenetic gene expressions.

Epigenetic gene expression makes changes to chemical groups in genes, essentially turning them on or off. I don't want to bog you down with all the technical elements. Just be aware that food, stress and environment, among other things, can and does alter your genes. There is a lot of info out there and it is fascinating.

Your Energy Can Affect Gene Expression

I have been talking a lot about energy so far. A big part of what this book's message is about is energy. We are all just energy after all. There happens to be yet another, energetic way to alter your genes.

There is a non-profit health organization called the HearthMath institute. "HeartMath Institute is committed to helping awaken the heart of humanity. We believe that when we align and connect our hearts and minds and connect with others, we awaken the higher mental, emotional and spiritual capacities that frequently lie dormant." This is straight from the about page on the HearthMath website. What I found interesting is their methods are very similar to mediation.

Magnetic Fields Are Powerful

Carlo Ventura, M.D., Ph.D., Editor-in-Chief of the World Journal of Stem Cells and professor at the University of Bologna in Italy. Discovered that by using magnetic field frequencies stem cells can be altered. Not only that, he says, "nonstem adult cells can be epigenetically reprogrammed backward to a state where they can eventually give rise to neural cells, cardiac cells, skeletal muscle cells or insulin-producing cells." Talk about malleability!

Drawing my own conclusions from this information. We can infer that everyday of our life we are changing and have the ability to manipulate our own gene expression. The secret is tapping into that magnetism. The

HeartMath Institute seems to have found one way to do exactly that. As mentioned already, genetic determinism is the traits you are born with. Epigenetics is signaling genes on and off.

Being A Victim Of Nature Or Controlling Your Health Destiny

Stem cell biologist and bestselling author Bruce Lipton, PhD says, "The difference between these two is significant because this fundamental belief called genetic determinism literally means that our lives, which are defined as our physical, physiological and emotional behavioral traits, are controlled by the genetic code," He further states, "This kind of belief system provides a visual picture of people being victims: If the genes control our life function, then our lives are being controlled by things outside of our ability to change them. This leads to victimization that the illnesses and diseases that run in families are propagated through the passing of genes associated with those attributes. Laboratory evidence shows this is not true."

Quantum Nutrients

Here is where energy comes in. HearthMath Institute calls this energy "Quantum Nutrients." According to Dr. Lipton, "When we have negative emotions such as anger, anxiety and dislike or hate, or think negative thoughts...we experience stress and our energy reserves are redirected." Researchers have found that human intentions can alter DNA strands using what HearthMath Institute refers to as heart coherence, "a beneficial state of mental, emotional and physical balance and harmony." Meditation, but more focused.

The heart generates a stronger electromagnetic field than the brain does. In one 2003 study, Modulation of DNA Conformation by Heart-Focused Intention by McCraty, Atkinson, Tomasino, it states, "Individuals capable of generating high ratios of heart coherence were able to alter DNA conformation according to their intention... Control group participants showed low ratios of heart coherence and were unable to intentionally alter the conformation of DNA."

What this means is that through thoughtful, heart centered intention, participants in this study were able to change DNA samples through focused intentions. These participants were able to alter their personal energetic signature and embed simple command messages inside of it. In turn changing their electromagnetic field into a sort of programming module that interacted with DNA strands. Specifically, they held DNA in a test tube in their hand and focused on unraveling the strands, and it worked.

Previously, I mentioned Robert Edward Grant. Remember he had made some discoveries implying that humans are made from binary code set into our DNA through frequencies. If our DNA can be created through energetic means then it can also be altered through the same. Which is what these studies have shown. It's all very fascinating when you start connecting the dots.

Serotonin Regulates Mood, Anxiety and Depression

You may not know that sugar is the most addictive legal substance in the world. Think about how your mood and energy levels change after consuming sugar, or during a prolonged absence of sugar in your diet. Not only that, sugar significantly affects serotonin levels. As I mentioned already, roughly 93% of your body's serotonin is produced in the gut.

Serotonin is a very important neurotransmitter that regulates mood, anxiety and depression. Most antidepressants work by blocking serotonin receptors. All of these factors combine to alter your personality and energetic signature.

When consuming sugar or corn syrup we are affecting serotonin production. That's why we get the sugar rush, and grumpy crash. By living in our guts, these corn syrup producing microorganisms could very well be altering our gene expression, affecting our fear response, mood, energy levels, electromagnetic signature, thinking and clarity. Sending craven signals to our brain to eat more foods with corn syrup in them.

How Corn Syrup, Food And Energy Are Altering Your DNA

Let's tie it all together. Extrapolating from above, we know that food, environment, and energy are able to alter human DNA expression. We also know that microorganisms in our gut can affect our thinking, mood, fear response and energy. We also know that our mood, thinking, and intentions can alter energy and our genes.

Corn syrup is produced using the waste products of bacteria and fungi. In the process of separating the α-amylase from the bacteria, and the γ-amylase from the fungi. It is almost certain that there is still DNA, bacteria and fungi (or spores) present in the solution used to manufacture the starches into corn syrup and the final product.

Even if, and this is a big if, the producers were able to completely remove all these bacteria and fungi. The process uses some of the most common forms available. Meaning you are likely ingesting and inhaling these same bacteria and fungi regularly. It's very possible these microorganisms are actively consuming sugars and/or fermenting carbohydrates and corn syrup in your gut, altering your well-being negatively.

Carbohydrates Are Fermentable Inside Our Gut

Sugar is not the only thing that can lead to fermentation in the gut. So can carbohydrates. In the US many breads contain corn syrup and/or sugar. Do you happen to eat a lot of bread, pasta and carbs? Ever take antibiotics? It's not just a theory that fermentation is happening in our guts.

A 46 year old man in the US was arrested for drunk driving, despite saying he hadn't drunk any alcohol. Yet, none would believe him, not his family or the doctors. After a variety of doctor visits he was finally diagnosed with Auto Brewery Syndrome (ABS).

This is when your body makes alcohol in your gut. The results are devastating. People with ABS have hallucinations, will act moody, aggressive, belligerent and paranoid. In this case doctors surmised, due to a previous injury he had been prescribed antibiotics and this threw off the bacterial balance in his gut. Which opened the door for those alcohol producing bacteria to thrive and take over.

The Balance Of Microflora In Our Gut Is More Important Than We Think

According to the CDC (Center for Disease Control) in America four out of five people are prescribed antibiotics each year and one out of three antibiotics prescriptions are unnecessary. Antibiotics are also contributing to the huge increase in allergies. Per the NIH (National Institute for Health), early life exposure to antibiotics increases the risk of eczema by as much as forty percent. Other studies have shown that the rise in antibiotic use has coincided with higher rates of asthma. Knowing this it is pretty easy to come to the conclusion. When we don't have full control of our gut health, we don't have full control of ourselves.

In my personal experience owning a kombucha brand for more than a decade. I received a lot of positive feedback from our clients. It was common to hear from people with skin problems, who said after drinking Pure Luck, their skin issues had cleared up. In another case. After drinking our kombucha regularly for a month, a man who had strong food allergies to seafood suddenly didn't have those same adverse effects anymore.

The most common feedback came from people with lethargy, IBS or constipation. Our kombucha always seemed to help ease or totally cure these symptoms. What is kombucha after all, but a symbiotic culture of beneficial yeasts and bacterias.

This is not to say you should go drink kombucha and it's going to cure you of all your ills. I only bring up these points to create the awareness that there is a lot more going on in our guts than we know. It's also important to be careful about the food and bacterial combinations we ingest.

Processed Foods Are Unnatural

It's not a stretch to say that all the processed foods, bacterias and sugars are affecting human health, mood, and thinking. There's also a very good chance they will also end up altering your genes, behavior and personality. I personally believe they are engineered this way.

Corn syrup and sugar are both highly fermentable. It's entirely realistic that one of both are fermenting in your gut reproducing GMO altered gene affected microbiota. I will go out on a limb and say the chance of all this happening is more likely than not. Not only that, the producers of these products know this.

The Hidden Truth

The sugar, tobacco, and oil companies hid research for decades showing they knew exactly the effects of their products on people and the environment. You have to consider that a company like Nestlé with 500 people working on the science of food will know a thing or two about what their products are capable of.

This is the nature of big business. How could you not be suspicious of giant global corporate conglomerates with hundreds of scientists working on ways to use food to alter gene expression? To keep you coming back for more. Of course it's not just Nestlé. The entire industry is built around maximizing profits and hooking customers. Corn syrup could just be one single example of the bio weapons being used against humans to create complacent addicts.

Natural Remedies Are Suppressed

On the other end of the spectrum there's a very simple weed that has so many components in it that are beneficial for human health. Its health applications have been known since at least the 1830s. Many of these same health benefits are backed up today by research.

The human body even has receptors, specifically to receive the components of this very plant. This weed is cannabis. Which as recently as the 1950s, grew wild in Brooklyn, NY. And is finally now legal in New York again. Cannabis has been a part of humanity since we have been humans. Only it was always called cannabis.

The term marihuana is associated with Mexicans who were immigrating to America in the early 1900s and smoking cannabis. This is why the architect of the illegalization movement changed the wordage. It helped to shape the public perception that only Black people, Mexicans, and Latinos were users. That man was Harry Anslinger, the first DEA commissioner.

Harry Anslinger's Aspirations

Harry Anslinger and the US government decided to wage a war that affected hundreds of millions of people, damaging societies around the world. The damage is still rippling almost one hundred years later. Yes, his main motivation was racism. It was also done with selfish interest to make himself more powerful. Even more interesting, if you look at the timing historically, the push to criminalize cannabis just so happens to coincide with the coming up of the pharmaceutical industry. A coincidence hard to deny.

Our Food System Is Political

The same thing can be said for our food system. It has been commercialized so much that it's become political. And it is political. The state of health and food in America and many other countries as well, is this way on purpose. The meat, dairy, and corn lobby in just the United States alone are a multi-trillion dollar force to reckon with. The United States is also one of the world's largest sugar producers.

If fight or flight is pre-installed firmware, what if our "second brain," our gut processor, has been hacked by modernity? A silent coup occurred unknowingly to us. These bad actors take up real estate in our gut just like the probiotic pirates do with the baby Mookie Wuuks in the fictional story in chapter 3.

These bad actors setup command and control stations. They hack the signals to our brain. Dulling the clarity of our thoughts, distracting our focus, affecting our decision making, and sending craving signals for more of their species and food sources.

It's All About The Messaging

As I already pointed out the majority of the serotonin is produced in the gut (93%). Some of serotonin's biological functions include modulating mood, cognition, reward, learning, memory, and numerous physiological processes. If we are consuming bio weapons—purposefully engineered to disrupt these processes—wouldn't it make sense. One, to target the gut and serotonin. And two, when we are caught up in daily survival, trusting our gut decisions, that we don't even realize the decision making process has been hacked?

I run these types of tests on myself all the time. I believe my gut instinct is very accurate and have trusted it all my life. And it's definitely shown up for me when I needed it most. I noticed when I am eating clean, exercising and mediating regularly my gut decisions are spot on. Almost as if I can predict the future. But when I'm tired and haven't been eating so clean or sleeping well. Often when I'm really busy or have been traveling a lot. My decision making becomes sub par.

How could a human know the messages have been hacked? Especially, if we have been consuming these foods and drinks from birth. If you think about it you have to ask. Who are we really? Have you ever even met your true self? Which makes me think of something. I did the Master Cleanse.

Which simply is fasting 10 days while drinking only lemon juice water with maple syrup and cayenne pepper. It's actually a delicious concoction. Fasting changed my personality completely. Not only that, my libido skyrocketed and my sense of smell became incredibly strong.

However, it is not an easy task to fast for ten days. And very much worth it if you can do it. I often think about Siddhartha when he fasts for 29 days in the book of the same name, written by Herman Hesse.

I mention fasting because it's a great way to restart your system. Just 3 days is enough to feel the benefits. You have to prepare for it properly. But if you have never fasted before and have the willpower to fast 10 days, you have the willpower to do anything. Resetting your gut system will recalibrate your taste buds too.

Cravings and moods are there to give a signal to buy something, to consume something. Go shopping, it will improve your mood. Eat that candy, it will make you feel better. Low on energy? Have some sugar or an energy drink. If you can control that urge. And eliminate it entirely. You are making progress.

Time For That Metaphorical Mental Dongle - Stop, Think, Question

There's no measure, context, or signals to say, "Wait a minute, eat more lactobacillus." "Eat more probiotics." We may not wonder why we are "feeling" and reacting a certain way. Mostly because we are probably too busy with the myriad of life related tasks and stress.

Living day to day humans just do as things come along, most of the time without very much thought or analysis. Why should a human think about these things? They have been living this way since birth. This is the only paradigm known. These are our cultures, and culture wars. The ones we have been trained to repeat.

Many don't think about processes and systems, or where the food they eat comes from, let alone how this food affects our bodies. How many people actually read the ingredients on the label? We just receive signals that tell us, "This tastes good." "This makes me feel better." Ohh I want to eat this! Cutting through the smokescreen is a lot of work if our guts have been hacked.

Masters and Servants

If the overlords keep humans busy enough with life, work, bills and the rules. If they keep the populace riled up with fear based media and hopped up on chemicals. Then most humans probably won't have time or energy to think or question. We'll just keep doing as we have always done, keep consuming as we are told to do—mind your lane. It is too much work to fight the system. The political gut is designed this way.

So humans end up craving and taking courses of action because they have been conditioned by the manufacturers and advertisers. Buying and consuming to lift their moods, or to get more energy, or to get that rush from the purchase. To feel gratified and better about ourselves, about our lives.

Humans are eating foods and drinks because the human brain via serotonin production and the gut has been hacked by corporations and governments. These institutions know fear, conspiracy, sugar, caffeine, fat, salt, alcohol, nicotine are addictive. They know how to pull strings, create addiction, and much, much more. How to make you feel crappy so you need something to feel happy.

Becoming Your Own Master

When I personally cut out everything and started meditating every day, my entire life changed. I stopped feeling the desire to consume like before. My favorite part is that now I am in control. I control my inputs. If I decide to have a cheat day it's a treat. And I know exactly what to expect. It was like kicking an addiction and becoming my own master. Of course I still have wants, but it's a different feeling when you are in control.

I desire to go snowboarding. Because I enjoy the clean, cold mountain air, the exhilarating physical experience and natural beauty of the mountains. I desire to travel more for my love of learning and seeing new things. I desire peace on Earth and for everyone to have food, shelter and clean water. Because there's really no need for life to be any other way. Especially in the United States, the richest nation on Earth.

Being Grateful And Content

There is a fine line between wants and desires. Most days I feel happy and grateful with the little I have and the most basic of foods. For example, I'll get excited looking forward to eating a ripe peach after my meal. It's such a delightful experience to live in the moment and savor the flavor, texture and aroma.

And on the days I am not feeling 100%, I am able to recognize what's going on. Never turning to consumption, alcohol, caffeine or sugar to make me feel better. I meditate longer, hit the gym, eat a mango, go for a run, a hike, a walk, or just lay on the bed staring at the ceiling daydreaming for 20-30 minutes.

The simple act of taking time for yourself will uplift your mood. Most of the time meditation alone is enough to make me feel connected and grateful. When I do feel down I try to compliment someone, have a positive interaction or do something good for someone else. Which always lifts me back up.

It is just like the HearthMath Institute says, when we align and connect our hearts and minds and connect with others, we awaken the higher mental, emotional, and spiritual capacities that frequently lie dormant. I really do feel content without consumption. And I can say from experience, I know what it is to not feel content, to feel that endless desire to fill deep holes of need.

Adaptability Without Need

This is not to say I don't need things to be a part of society. Of course I typed this book on a laptop. I have to wear clothes. I love to travel. I sleep in a bed with pillows and organic sheets. My point is that I don't need these things. They are privileges. We used to live in caves!

It was only 30 years ago that laptops became a necessity and only 15 for iPhones. Overall, I've reduced my consumption by 95%. An added benefit is all the money saved and better experiences had. I love fashion and dressing nicely, but at the same time I wore the same clothes with holes in them for two years while I wrote this book.

When I lived in Japan, I slept on a futon on the floor. In Thailand when there were only cold showers or no AC, I adapted. When I first moved to France. I slept on the smallest single bed for 2 years. My feet were dangling off the bottom, but I always felt happy to have a bed, roof and food. Even if there's only rice to eat, only eat rice and enjoy the singular flavor. There's probably soy sauce somewhere. I'll for sure look.

When I don't have to be on the computer, I am grateful not to have to use one. This state of freedom exists. Technology, too many possessions, needs, consumption and social media creates a form slavery. Always having to update the software, check your emails, keep track of passwords, be afraid of viruses and hacks, manage subscriptions, get the newest version, craven consumption for something.

If you can bring yourself back to natural you will find context and your true self. You will be able to eject the hackers. I successfully ejected the hackers and everyone can also do the same. I will never tell you it is easy though. If you want to feel good it takes a concerted effort.

Recognizing Your Messaging System Has Been Hacked

These hacked messages become a sort of self reinforcing echo chamber. Humans trust their feelings because we are conditioned to do so. Since the hackers are hungry they order room service. Normally, in a natural state these cravings will be fruits, nuts or greens. I get these messages daily. I crave salad, an apple, a banana or pomelo. Best part is I eat them, feel great and there's no crash. Just feeling great.

But on the hackers craven message board, it is corporation one and corporation two. Because they know what makes you tick more than you know what makes you tick. This is a very huge advantage. Why would you let them have this massive advantage over you?

The Strength Of Awareness

Politicians, kings, brands, and advertisers have known about human physiology and psychology for a very long time. They actively use these traits against us. Being strong mentally is actually much more energy and work than just toughness as most people think of it.

This toughness entails a lot of understanding about food, methods, and business practices. Governments, history, and society. Learning about how other cultures in different countries live. Experiencing those ways of being first hand. Growing perspective to gain better contextual understanding.

This is homework that involves reading about scientific studies and doing some research. Digging for information. Cutting through all the misinformation and fluff. Learning all the things they won't teach you in school. Asking a lot of questions.

Sounds like a lot of work right? It is, without a doubt, a significant undertaking. Not one that is unachievable. Life is long! Just by reading this book I hope you are already gaining knowledge and new understanding. Maybe you even have already started asking more questions of yourself. Baby steps are all you need. Just keep moving forward.

It Has To Be A Conscious Choice

Working toward this freedom is also bodybuilding the right bacteria compositions inside (and outside) of our bodies. This includes things like creams, shampoo, soap, detergent and makeup. Sleeping right and making informed choices when grocery shopping and eating out.

Being annoying to anyone who doesn't want to share the facts. Reading labels and living in places where the environment is less toxic, where access to quality organic food is easier. You have to choose this life. For some this choice may be impossible. But it's not hopeless. Each step forward is progress in the right direction.

It's Work Worthy Of Collective Participation

Work as we define it in the 21st century usually involves some sort of monetary payment. This type of work does not. Yet, it will save you money. And if it is quantified by happiness, quality of life, and fewer doctor visits. Plus, it brings about a kinder, happier, healthier, more connected populace. If those are the benefits, then surely this work could be a sort of investment in the future and worthy of everyone's participation for the benefit of society, humanity, climate, and the planet. And your children.

Let's call it a quantum-directional workout. Humans already consume proteins and aminos to build muscle, just need to take it a step further. Our food and thinking is tied to our gut health and patterns of experiences we register emotionally.

As newborns we inherit our mother's microbiota. As soon as we come into the world we build on that by consuming food and drink given to us by our parents. Each house in each city has a different micro-biome. The living microbiome is all around us. We are its unknowing servants.

If we become aware of this and cultivate a positive living microbiome in our home, on our bodies, and inside our gut, then we are able to control it before it controls us. When we control our energetic signature we control our destiny. The first step is gaining the knowledge that this must be done. You are already gathering momentum.

CHAPTER EIGHT

Re-Prioritize

Everything, everywhere around us, all the space is energy. Again, to be exact, 99.99999% energy. Only .00001% is matter. In a vacuum, energy cannot be removed. Energy is omnipresent. What is energy? Many different things manifest in different shapes and forms.

Plants Can Feel, Hear And Remember

There are studies which have shown plants are susceptible to a person's energy and know when they enter the room. In another study published in Entomology Today in 2014 the researchers showed that plants can hear and remember.

These researchers played the sounds of a caterpillar munching on leaves from a tape recorder and the plants responded by producing chemical defenses. "What is remarkable is that the plants exposed to different vibrations, including those made by a gentle wind or different insect sounds that share some acoustic features with caterpillar feeding vibrations, did not increase their chemical defenses," Professor Rex Cocroft said.

"Previous research has investigated how plants respond to acoustic energy, including music," said Heidi Appel, a research scientist. "However, our work is the first example of how plants respond to an ecologically relevant vibration. We found that feeding vibrations signal changes in the plant cells' metabolism, creating more defensive chemicals that can repel attacks from caterpillars." There is much more intelligence on this planet than just ours.

Our Food Is Energy Beyond What Is Defined As Calories

In addition to nutrition and intelligence, becoming aware that food has energy is important. Food is also 99.99999% energy and .00001% matter. Humans must consider the way foods are handled, treated, and grown. The attention, or not, paid to it and the care in which it is handled. The microbial content of the soil, the history of the soil, the climate and stress of the plant, the farmers and planet. The happiness and virility of the plant, the quality of the air it breathes.

How could these things not affect the nutrition, energy content, quality, and taste? A human will be less healthy, and more prone to illness should they be raised on a meager diet, exposed to dangerous chemicals, high stress, and starved of nutrients. It's not just a plant. We are what we eat.

Stress Is Stress, In All Life Forms

Why would this idea be so radical or different for any living thing, plant, insect, or animal? Fear causes the release of chemicals. The release of chemicals causes fear. More stress impacts healthy functioning.

In animals these hormones have been shown to taint the flavor of the meat and cheese. Why wouldn't this be applicable to a plant? Plants are living and they communicate with each other. Maybe humans don't speak plant language—though these days there are some scientists who are learning to speak plant.

The logical train of thought gives cause to infer the same, as with all other living things. They are still 99.99999% energy. We have an intuitive sense that a healthy plant will possess more nutrition and taste.

Chef Dan Barber

Chef Dan Barber of Blue Hill Farm and Stone Barns has proven this. He has been named one of America's 100 most influential people in Time magazine. He has also received several James Beard awards and given Ted talks. In his Ted talks he highlights how sustainability actually creates better tasting food. I recommend watching his Ted talks. They are very interesting. He is referred to in The Gothamist as a "chef-thinker," exploring taste, sustainability, and meaning in food.

For one of his experiments he partnered with some local farms in upstate New York. What they found is nothing short of remarkable. Healthier plants—as defined by more microbial diversity within the soil they grow in—had fuller, more flavorful profiles and higher nutritional content.

Turns Out It's All About The Microbiome

The microbiome in the soil interacts with the roots of the plant. These microscopic life forms make nutrients bio-available to the plant. In much the same way, bacteria in the human gut makes nutrients available for the human body.

Healthier soil is defined by more diversity of microbes, in turn facilitating more availability of nutrients for plant uptake. This made the plants produce taste better and have more nutrition. It's so very simple, let nature work for us. Nature knows the way, having been around much longer than humans have. There are a couple more studies that further these ideas.

Energy Is Omnipresent

Scientists in Europe made cheese from goat's milk. For this study. They herded goats into a pristine mountain pasture, full of herbs and grasses.

In an area with no known predators. The goats were encircled with a natural wood fence. When the time came, the scientists milked the goats and made cheese. Then they tested for stress hormones and other related compounds.

The experiment was repeated. Same goats, same pasture. This time the scientists replaced the wood with an electric fence to contain the goats. What they discovered was that the goats, when enclosed by an electric fence, produced milk with more stress hormones. This resulted in the cheese being described as having "off flavors". When compared to the first cheese made when the goats were enclosed by a wooden fence.

The goats therefore must be able to sense, or hear the electric field created by the fence, which must give them stress. Birds use Earth's energy field, or magnetoreception to navigate. Every living plant and animal, including humans, are tapped into this field of energy all around us. It's why sometimes some people give you a bad feeling. Energy is the basic building block of life.

Humans Have The Same Sense Of Perception

Have you ever been to New York City? As a resident for twenty years it was very obvious to me that humans are able to detect this energy. As soon as you cross the Hudson river from New Jersey, the energy in Manhattan is very strong and present enough to feel it.

Humanity may have dulled their overt perception to lesser energies. Yet, this doesn't rule out the probability. We are much more connected than we are able to recognize. Not only that, but humans are actually able to fine tune this connection, to gain a better reception to the energy. To be able to use and communicate with the energy that surrounds us and creates our physical being.

I'm sure you can think of an experience in your life where you had thought transference with a close friend, lover, or relative. There are studies that prove we can read other peoples minds. From couples "thinking in sync" to being able to feel it when someone is looking at you, and more.

Once we fine tune the reception, we are able to receive the messages more accurately. To bring this into a more overt subconscious behavior. I believe the first step is to remove the toxins dulling our sensors by actively changing our diet and lifestyle.

The Cheese Nun

Perhaps my favorite type of natural versus unnatural stories is that of the Cheese Nun in Bethlehem, PA, with a PhD in Microbiology. She was able to successfully prove to the USDA that the use of man made, stainless steel cheese molds results in mitigation of beneficial bacterial strains. Simultaneously, stainless steel use promoted the growth of unwanted e-coli bacterial strains.

On the other hand, natural wood cheese molds created better tasting, more balanced microbial diverse cheese that limited the growth of e-coli. The American federal government wants to force all food production to use stainless steel for everything. Having worked in the food industry for a very long time. I have experience with this first hand.

Using Nature As Our Guide

Instead of being forced to do things in an unnatural way we should trust in and let nature be our guide. This is called biomimicry. Nature has had billions of years of trial and error and already knows the best ways. We simply need to enmesh ourselves with observation, connect, and follow nature's lead.

The constant need to bend nature to our way is short sighted and out of balance. Humans actually are very adaptable. Wouldn't it seem more efficient and responsible to bend ourselves to the natural world around us? To love, cherish, and connect with it. After all, it sustains our species.

Our ancestors did this for millennia. I don't mean that humans need to live in grass or mud huts, although there have been some interesting modern architectural works using mud and hay. My point is that humans have sent men to the moon and can watch videos online of Mars! Humanity has the intelligence, resources, and technology to enmesh with the natural world around us. Do we have the will to use it sustainably to create more understanding and a better quality of life for all? Easy, quick, and greedy triumph in our current paradigm.

Instead of changing ourselves to live in harmony with the planet, humans have created industry on such a scale that we are changing the course of the natural world, the climate, and the planet. We are driving species to extinction and destroying the very systems we rely on to sustain us. This is just so hard to comprehend, all in the name of money, control, and power.

Time For A New System

Maybe there are simply too many humans and politicians to control. Maybe then, instead of enforcing a one way system of taking of which we all partake. Society should instead demand a self reinforcing cycle of health, wealth, and excellent quality of life for everyone. Who could argue against this? There must be some who do argue against it.

Yet, it seems selfish and angry to want others to fail and be miserable. What would this new way look like? It is absolutely possible. Do not let anyone tell you this is not possible. A simple shift in humanity's collective mindset. From me, the ego, the quick, easy, and greedy. Unto us the compassionate and collective, the needless, caring and thoughtful, kind and flexible. These kinds of sentences always sound corny. But could you imagine how good life would be if a shift like this took place?

A replacement of values will open up a mindset of abundance instead of one of scarcity. How could this change? Simply by changing our diets and lifestyles. Rejecting processed foods, business as usual and rejecting mindless consumption. Teaching every child to meditate starting from a very young age. Eliminating the millions of unnecessary products, chemical additives and learning to be content with less things and more with better experiences. We could shift the economy, because if there was suddenly less consumption where would all the jobs be?

What Is Valuable?

Ideas of what is valuable need to be redefined. We must place value on the environment and human connectedness and well-being. We must spend more time creating the necessary, instead of the superfluous. This is already beginning to happen in some parts of the world, namely Amsterdam.

In 2021 the Dutch have been rethinking business as usual, implementing an extremely simple economic theory dreamt up by a woman named Kate Raworth called Doughnut Economics. She consults all over the world and wrote a book of the same name, Doughnut Economics. The book asks us to look at economies and society in a different way, using the word doughnut and bringing the idea of round to mind.

Doughnut Economics

Kate Raworth places value on what is important within the doughnut. That which is unimportant resides outside of it. Rather than putting emphasis on endless growth as measured by GDP (gross domestic product), the emphasis is based on thriving in balance with the world and society around us as measured by quality of life.

She argues, quite successfully, humanity must change the way economics is taught and re-think where we place value. The current curriculum involved in the teaching of economics in Universities worldwide relies on a very outdated model. I recommend her book, it is a very easy read.

Entrenched Interests

Naturally, the current system is rigged against this. Politicians, billionaires, and the elite prefer things to stay the way they are. They are the winners in this society. They will surely use their massive advantages, connections, and resources to fight against anything that changes the status quo. Don't forget human psychology dictates that humans will fight for something that is being lost, much harder than fighting to gain something new.

So the powerful will no doubt fight very hard against anything that costs them money because many are cheap; cheap minded, and cheap in the pocket. They like profits at the top, people at the bottom. In order to make change, we must all collectively wake from the politically and chemically induced stupor. Stand up and hit these humans where it hurts. Destroy their profits.

Stop Consuming To Destroy Business As Usual

In chapter 17 I've made a list of things I personally do not consent to, yet really have no power over. Collectively we all must take a stand at once. One way to do this could simply be to stop going to work at jobs we dislike for terrible pay. While the CEOs pay themselves handsomely. We could also stop buying mindlessly and vote with our money, only buying the most basic of necessities.

If five million people were to decide to strike at once. Just by simply not consuming, not driving their cars, or working at their jobs, not going on social media, not watching TV for one week. Instead just sit home and relax, learn to meditate, talk to your neighbors, sit outside, read a book, and turn off your devices. This would send a message.

Businesses couldn't fire five million people all at once. One peaceful act of civil disobedience could stop everything in its tracks. If this message isn't loud enough, if they fight back. Then hit them harder. Grow the movement to ten million people for two weeks.

This is the most simple form of peaceful protest. Just sit at home. Do not spend any money, consume nothing, save money and refuse to work. Until this system breaks and changes. With this type of mobilization, the elites, corporations, and politicians will have to listen.

Corruption And Fallibility

One of the biggest issues humanity faces is that humans are so easily fallible and corrupted. Thus far, humanity is heading down a dark and dangerous path where the only outcome will be our extinction. These are not my worlds either. These are the words of experts in extinction studies. These experts say if humans do not change immediately, humanity will cease to exist, in short order.

Humans are killing our host, the Earth. If the systems of the Earth become unstable—and they are already, clearly showing signs of instability—then our entire existence is at stake. What do we have to lose by taking action? What more of a wake up call is needed?

Look around at the climate. We are frogs in a bowl with the burner on. Slowly cooking to death. Slowly poisoning ourselves to death. Dying from cancer and disease. We don't have to choose this path. But we do have to stand up and stop acting like entitled, lazy, egocentric, greedy monkeys.

Embrace Balance and Peace Of Mind

There exists a much better paradigm right in front of us. All we need to do is shift our thinking and embrace the importance of balance in thinking, living, existence, and environment. We are so in excess right now, so unbalanced. So many things that humans produce and consume are simply just not necessary to our survival or needs.

Most products are simply a means to and an end for a very select few. Not only that, but these massive excesses are directly leading to our decline and furthering the future of indebted servitude. The more chaos and broken the system. The more power those who control the systems gain over the rest.

The Plastic Epidemic

Take plastics for example. Microplastics have been found in the feces of babies and adults. On Mt. Everest and in the deepest oceans. They have even been found in the human bloodstream, bowel, lungs and testicles.

In a new study published in December of 2021, which the scientists are saying they need more time to confirm. Preliminary data shows that microplastics in our environment are causing IBS (Irritable Bowel Syndrome). The study found that people with IBS had 50% more micro plastics in the colon than people without IBS.

Micro-plastics are pervasive. They are in our tap and bottled water, our toothpaste. In our food and air. They have been found in the most remote places on Earth. They are killing fish, animals, and humans. Yet, armed with this knowledge. Nothing changes and it is still business as usual.

On January 1st, 2022, France banned the use of plastic wrapping for vegetables. This is a great start but far from enough. In January of 2022, at the supermarket in America, I found individually wrapped prunes in a plastic bag. Who needs individually wrapped prunes? Meaning one single prune, wrapped in plastic. About twenty of them. In a bag made of plastic!

Who Sells Us Convenience?

Corporations are selling you the idea of quick and easy convenience. This way you have more time to work at your job or do other consumption related tasks. Convenience makes humans subservient and lazier to make an effort to do things for themselves. This is a self reinforcing cycle.

For me personally the more lazy I become, the more lazy I want to be. I am sure I am not alone here. This is the very opposite of what must happen. Big business knows that easy and lazy is big money. Because they are the ones filling our foods with chemicals and nasty stuff to make us feel this way. They are the ones asking us to work longer shifts for less pay and buy convenience food, fast food, TV dinners and apparently individually wrapped prunes.

Corporations Are Not Altruistic

What is being done to stop this? As of now nothing. Business as usual precludes change. Change costs effort to the human and corporation. If consumers are not demanding change, then surely there will be no investment on the part of the corporations.

Corporations prefer to spend money buying back shares of their stock and increasing the shareholder value of the already wealthy instead of investing in upgrades and advancement. This is not just me saying this. This is the reality of what is happening presently in corporate America.

With a very minor exception, the vast majority of micro-plastics and plastics are made from petroleum. These plastics don't degrade for hundreds of years. Humans live in a petroleum society, even the US Dollar is called the "Petro-Dollar." Many critics of change fear monger, that the economy will crash if humans change from being petroleum people.

I often wonder, do these same people think about their children and grandchildren? Do they think about what we will do if the Earth becomes uninhabitable? Of course they must. That's why the billionaire class wants to colonize Mars. "To save humanity."

So they can send the rich and their children into escape pods from Earth when it becomes uninhabitable. Do you think the average citizen will be invited? Only if they need some slave labor. Who wants to live on Mars anyway? It's not going to be as pleasant as living on Earth. Why are we not focusing on saving the place where we live now? Because that would destroy the profits. This is upside-down thinking at its finest.

Chemical Pollution Has Crossed a "Planetary Boundary"

In January 2022, The Guardian reported on a new study. The study concludes that chemical pollution has crossed a "planetary boundary," the point at which human-made changes to the Earth push it outside the stable environment of the last 10,000 years.

The title of the article, Chemical Pollution has Passed Safe Limit for Humanity. It reads: "Plastics are of particularly high concern, they said, along with 350,000 synthetic chemicals including pesticides, industrial compounds and antibiotics." Basically, these scientists are saying the same thing I have been saying for many decades.

"Chemical pollution threatens Earth's systems by damaging the biological and physical processes that underpin all life." The question is, what are we going to do about it? I wrote a report about this in high school. In the 1990s! Nothing has changed. The problem has only doubled and tripled and quadrupled.

Change The Existing Power Structures

How could humanity change the system if the system is rigged and controlled by big oil? By 1% of the population? Many of the billionaire class want to depopulate the Earth. This is also not my theory. They have no interest in saving lives.

In my opinion they are actively working to kill off as many humans as they can. When looking around it's not a hard conclusion to draw. These very same people have convinced humanity that without them humanity is screwed.

If the politicians are controlled by the oil companies and corporations. Then they don't have the will to do what is right. Either way, everyday humans are getting the short end of the stick! We have to re-prioritize. Change is not happening fast enough.

Humans just do what is easy, throwing our hands in the air. "Easy" is common. "Easy" is all humans think we can do. The same statement is being said over and over. Every day, "What can I do?" I am just one person. It is too much to deal with on top of work and stress and the kids.

Easy Is Common When You Are Stressed And Tired

At the same time, these very same corporations are creating products of convenience which they will happily sell to us. This way people have more time to spend with burdensome regulations. More time to spend working to make the 1% richer. Complacent, tired, and worn out humans are easy to manipulate. Tired humans search for what is easy.

When people are slowed down from their food. And their busy and stressed out work schedule. Everyday dealing with bills, life, illness, social media, and society—too often looking for something to pick up their mood and give them temporary happiness and energy to keep up with daily life—then of course these same humans won't have time to think or question the system. Never mind attempting to elicit change. This is why the gut is political. The system is upside-down purposefully. It's meant to keep up at our wits' edge.

Groupthink Controls Us

I want to go into more detail about the psychological effects of group-think. Simply put, humans take on the views of others in a group to avoid confrontation. Even though these very same people may not agree internally, they will still act and agree externally. And social media supercharges group thinking.

Many humans may never even recognize this dynamic is at work or what truly feeling mentally free from groupthink is like. Never knowing what it's like to feel healthy and strong both mentally and physically. It's so much work to eat healthy, exercise, read all the ingredients and think for ourselves. To speak our mind and deal with the consequences. To research all the names of the additives. Learn the various detrimental side effects. Cook meals at home from locally purchased ingredients. To act differently from what everyone else is doing and say no to people.

The Design Reinforces Escapism

Most people want to escape their life and daily stresses. So they resort to alcohol, pain killers, antidepressants, and pharmaceuticals. It is much easier to pop a pill or open a bottle. Of course the system is designed this way. If people are so depressed with their life, they have to take an antidepressant to make them happy. Do you think the people on antidepressants will have the cognizance of mind to fight the system? I doubt it.

The government and corporations love when you take anti-depressants. When you pop pharmaceuticals and believe their every word. They know you will be a good, compliant little sheep. How could a human be anything else when hooked on pills waiting to get the next refill?

Why Is Sugar Legal But Not Cocaine?

What's the difference between cocaine and sugar? One is legal and can be grown in the United States as a cash crop. They are both just as addictive and have similar effects on the brain and dopamine levels.

According to studies done at Queensland University of Technology by neuroscientist and Professor, Selena Bartlett, "It (sugar) has also been shown to repeatedly elevate dopamine levels which control the brain's reward and pleasure centers in a way that is similar to many drugs of abuse including tobacco, cocaine and morphine. We have also found that as well as an increased risk of weight gain, animals that maintain high sugar consumption and binge eating into adulthood may also face neurological and psychiatric consequences affecting mood and motivation." The knowledge is right here hiding in plain sight.

The NIH agrees with these findings. The key point, sugar affects mood and motivation. Next time you are at the supermarket look at the nutrition panels on everyday items. When a 4oz. yogurt contains twenty grams of sugar. Now you know why. Not only does it motivate you to buy it again, but also when you are not high on the dopamine rush you get depressed, angry and lazy.

Dr James DiNicolantonio says, "When you look at animal studies comparing sugar to cocaine, even when you get the rats hooked on IV cocaine, once you introduce sugar, almost all of them switch to the sugar." Need I say more? I will in chapter 10.

It simply seems impossible for many people in this paradigm to fight the mental and physiological warfare. To create the presence of mind and willpower to make meaningful change for themselves. Humanity is thus trapped in a world built upside-down on purpose.

Turn Off The Money Flow

The paradigm has got to be changed. Humanity desperately needs big thinkers with willpower in positions of power. However, power mostly seems to entice those with corrupt intent. Firstly, it's more than time to take the money out of politics. There should be no campaign donations. No lobbying, no dark money groups. No connections whatsoever between the moneyed, the corporations, big business, the politicians and bodies that regulate business and food. I understand this is *huge* ask.

The laws should be so strict that even the most minute appearance of corruption or bribery will mean a very long stint in jail. Honesty needs to be placed above all else and political speech outlawed. Let's call it what it is really, lying. The critics are crying but free speech! Politicians must be held to a standard of honesty. No false advertising! If I lie on my resume. More often than not when the company finds out I'll be fired. Why doesn't this apply to elected officials? All they do is lie, and call it "political speech."

Having a system of honesty and trust will set an entirely new tone for citizens. To see a completely different set of examples and will directly alter society and return trust. But politicians don't want trust, they want you to be cynical. They want lying to be normalized.

This is better for corruption, easier even. We can see what's happening now in the political world. Look how the leaders are leading and in what direction. Look how corrupt influence spreads. If one person with a huge voice keeps pushing followers to be like them the corruption only grows.

Leading By Positive Example

Leading by example has to come from within power. Many political leaders right now have no interest in setting positive examples because it's better for them to have humans divided. The old saying "divide and conquer" is not just a saying. It's actively playing out right now.

We must change to a taxpayer funded political system. If citizens want to make tax deductible political donations that is great. These donations will go into one pool and be split evenly between candidates. This would open up the field to people who are not solely millionaires and billionaires.

There must be requirements, psychological evaluations and rigorous due diligence. The same as there is already for any high level position. This is a job, a very important job. They work for the citizens. The application process must be treated as so. How can a criminal lose the right to vote, but still be eligible to work as an elected official? Of course because politicians make the laws. They don't want to place any restrictions on themselves. Self regulation doesn't work with corporations and it surely doesn't work in politics. There should be a system of laws, not written by politicians, that are created specifically to regulate politicians.

The study and application of politics must only be for people who are actually interested in true "public service." The argument against this will be that this system will put our country at risk by having less sophisticated people in government. I think we already have many, very unsophisticated, selfish people in politics.

This will remove the ineptitude, the nepotism. The self serving, back scratching and corrupt influence of those who only care about money and power. Who wish to maintain their power and corruption at all costs. It can't remain that only the rich and powerful are able to be political leaders—such a system will forever benefit the few over the many.

The political party system must also be eliminated. Including even affiliation. Just individual people and their ideas. The affiliation system sets people apart into tribal thinkers. It creates division. It also allows for too much control over individual members through money, reprisals and bullying.

Change Begets Change

When the political and the economic models are changed from endless growth, self servitude and GDP. To place value on the environment, well-being, and societal benefit. There will be less will from those with corrupt intent—those who only care about big business and the moneyed class—to seek positions of power.

Of course the critics will say I am an idealist. The argument against this is that China or Russia or those other countries will take control of the world stage. Have you seen these countries' behavior lately? I don't think anyone is going to be looking up to these countries for some time.

America has been a leader for a very long time. I have traveled to twenty-seven counties and lived in four different countries. And will state from experience. The professionalism, innovation and idealism of America is unrivaled.

Yet, presently, America's influence has been waning . Precisely because of corruption and ineptitude. I wager that if the populations in other countries see how America is changing. How Americans are rising up against inequality, they too may rise up to make similar changes. Once again American influence will grow.

There Is Currency In A Strong Society

I'm not saying we have to decrease our strength as a nation. I am saying we have to increase our strength as a society. We must change the focus from greed, tribalism and power. The old way is failing and will certainly end badly.

Those that wield power today will die tomorrow. There is a new generation of humans and thinkers with new priorities already coming of age. It's not if, it is only when. Let's speed up the process by taking action now and laying the groundwork for a better future.

Money Should Never Equal Votes

We have the power to bring lobbying online. For every single person to access it with equal and anonymous power. People must demand that lobbying in its current state be made illegal. Lobbying the government is each human's right, not only the right of the rich. In the current system, dollars are equal to votes. Giving the wealthy more votes, as the US Supreme Court has ruled. This must be changed.

In true representative society, each person's voice carries the same weight. When citizens remove the money, power, and corrupt influence. Only then will we see people running for higher office with true and good intentions. Instead of a race to the bottom, it will be a race to the top.

Spurring those going into politics to perform duties truly as a public service instead of the self serving practice it is now. Politicians are not, and should never be treated as celebrities. We must demand change today. Yet, none of those in power now will be receptive to these changes. Something must happen to tear down these systems. Business as usual will surely see our decline. It already is.

Silver Linings

I think in some small ways the COVID pandemic has awakened people. The silver lining to all the death and craziness was time to sit and think. To recenter goals and needs, focusing on what is inside ourselves. Only we must not solely focus on ourselves. We must focus on the collective, seizing the day.

It's not We The People want freedom to do what we want. To be lawless. To tread all over others. It's We The People want freedom from the corruption and malfeasance that our current political and business as usual system embodies. Freedom to breathe clean air. Drink clean water. Eat food without chemicals and addictive additives. To be free to love and express our true selves. Not what the government and corporations want us to be.

Re-prioritize Your Thinking

Humanity must push back with our voices, actions, and minds. There are many who say they like these things. Let's keep it this way. These are addicted humans who have convinced themselves they need things to stay the same because change is scary and requires thought, learning and work.

Humans are addicted to easy, fast, and 'me' thinking. Afraid of change, afraid of the perceived loss of endless products available to them. Because of the need for things to fill those holes in themselves. This need goes away when you clear your body of the bad bacterias. To be a part of the collective is selflessness. Humans can still be free, while being natural and a collective. The freedom I speak of is significantly much freer than we are now. Humans just don't know it yet.

Cut The Fat

It's time to cut the fat. This will require some small sacrifices. Pushing back against the toxicity of greed, power, easy, 'me' thinking. If the collective forcibly breaks down the guardrails to change the discussion. Taking a stand and only buying and supporting what is necessary. We will make positive changes.

This is what being selfless is, not being selfish. Humans must learn to reject the easy. The convenient, chemical laden foods. Reject excess consumption, destruction of the environment. The endless purchasing of meaningless products that ultimately become waste. Humans must be the change they want to see in the world. We must be that change in ourselves first. Humanity has to pull together for the benefit of everyone.

Listen And Love

Right now the politicians are purposefully pushing people apart. But we must come together and help each other. Listening, speaking and opening our minds. Groupthink is very strong. So individually each human must take part and share the ideas of selflessness with their friends and neighbors. Just as negativity, fear, and complaining are contagious, so is hope, selflessness, joy, positivity and love.

You will feel good when you act this way. It's not just a cheesy statement, it is in our nature. Get addicted to that good feeling. The feeling of giving and inspiration. If you do it, your friends and peers will follow. And their friends and peers.

In advertising, the highest sales per hit are made on the recommendation from a friend. These recommendations can be as much as 90% effective. If each human spreads the word collectively for all to see, then it is possible to light a fire of change.

Stop Acting Like Monkeys

What is profit without the environment? If the planet dies so do we. Do you want your children to suffer needlessly because we were too lazy, too divided to act now? To be human, humanity needs to stop acting like monkeys and evolve to be actual intelligent beings.

Buckminster Fuller said "You never change things by fighting the existing reality. To change something, build a new model that makes the existing model obsolete." If everyone likes the world we live in and is healthy, happy and prosperous, then clearly that would be a paradigm to be adopted quickly.

However, right now, poll after poll shows, the vast majority say we are headed in the wrong direction. Then why are humans actually fighting so hard against changing direction? Rather than just changing direction. We keep fighting against our own best interests. Because we have been tricked into being angry haters instead of loving, kind neighbors.

Socialism Is A Code Word

What I have described above will be criticized as Socialism. Political parties rail against the boogeyman of "Socialism." What if we redefine the code? Socialism is just a code word used to scare us away from doing what's in our best interests. To keep the wealthy in power.

It triggers already forged, reflexive mental responses which are set purposefully like traps. If you are a person who doesn't want a hand to get up, that's fine. But you should not force your will, your way, on others who do want and need a hand. Just like you want to have a choice not to be tread on, so should others have the same choice not to be tread on by you.

Humans must rethink our core ideas of value, setting a baseline for every being. Humanity has the power, money, and technology to do it. It is simply a matter of will. Every human on this planet needs water, food, clean air, basic healthcare, somewhere to live and go to the bathroom. We can all agree on this. There's no waffling on these necessities.

Reprogram The Code Into Living Environment

Let's call this a "Living Environment" instead of Socialism. Rename this way of thinking, the Living Environment. Mentally associating positivity, wealth generation, social connections, crime reduction and kindness with the moniker, Living Environment.

No one is going to tax you 50% for a living environment. No one is going to make you take handouts if you don't need or want them. And no one is going to take handouts away from those who do need and want them. With no strings attached. The government is already giving huge sums of handouts to the corporations in the form of subsidies and tax breaks. Why can't taxpayer money be used to benefit the citizenry?

Removing the constant need for survival thinking will free people's minds to be more creative, innovative, happier, and healthier. This, in general, will lead people to focus on what they like, are interested in, and are good at. Redirecting the anger and resentment.

If humans are less stressed everyday about paying rent and putting food on the table this will free up mental space and energy. Creating new thought patterns and removing the survivalist mindset, nudging people to work more sustainably. Starting to do "work" that is more fulfilling for them. Freeing up more time to focus on building up themselves.

Repurpose Subsidies

We could totally redefine what pay is. What it means to be alive. If governments were to simply use the subsidies they give to the oil companies—not to mention all the other superfluous industries—and instead give every citizen earning less than x dollars per year some form of monthly stipend. Or as I lay out in a later chapter, a blockchain based token. We would be well on our way to a better society.

The companies that receive government subsidies are already making billions of dollars in profits, they don't need our tax dollars too! Why is the government giving corporations our money which they don't need? Instead of using your tax dollars to better your life!?

One problem for the elite with this system is that they will have a hard time finding the workers to do their crappy jobs. Another is it will be harder to divide people if they are happier, healthier, wealthier and thinking more clearly. That is the catch. It will also mean less political donations from big business!

That is why you will constantly hear the drumbeat of Socialism. Socialism is bad, they will tax you 80%. You will have to support all those freeloaders. Don't let these complainers trick you with the fake fear mongering. They are the freeloaders! They don't want to lose their subsidies.

There's no need for raising taxes. The only need is to make sure the wealthy pay their fair share. And the corporations don't get any charity they certainly don't need. I will lay out in greater detail how bad the subsidy situation is later on.

The Positive Effects Are Undeniable

There are already studies that prove the positive effects of a Living Environment. In Hudson, NY they have been providing a small number of people with just $500 a month. Guaranteed income, they call it. The results so far are being said to "reverse 'history of judgment' on people in poverty." The first year's data include increased social connections and more happiness. Employment rates among recipients more than doubled! People were left to make their own financial decisions. They felt empowered to think beyond day to day expenses and actually plan for the future.

This is moving from a scarcity mindset to an abundance mindset. In this case it only cost $500 a month, per person. The benefits of this on a massive scale will most certainly outweigh the financial costs. They already have systems like this in place in Europe. It's not some far off concept.

There is just too much inefficient and frankly stupid spending done in the government because politicians and giant corporations are way too close. The focus is all about the upside-down world for them. The government funnels the money from the taxpayers to the already wealthy. The legalized corruption is insane.

The Mental Burden Is All To Real

Other systems that need to be changed are benefits structures like SNAP (food stamps). These are highly regimented, tested, and bureaucratic. Which is mentally painful and demeaning if you are already poor. They don't help your body as much as they hurt your mind. It is not possible to exist in today's society without money. This is so obvious and basic. If you do not have money this affects thinking, self worth, and decision making.

Personally, I know this experience very well. There was a time when I went through a rough patch. I was homeless and broke in NYC. I can speak directly from experience. Every decision becomes based on money, even riding the subway.

Many times I had to resort to jumping the turnstile simply because I didn't have the fare. And this is a crime which can lead to even more fines and problems. It is a no win situation and is so painful to live this way. It scars the mind and is not easy to recover.

The Always Wealthy Will Never Be Objective

Since only the rich and super rich make our laws and run the government. These people are incredibly out of touch. Mostly, they don't care about regular people. Most will never understand the psychological mind state of the working classes.

I suspect most very wealthy people think they are above everyone else. Often referring to the working poor and the poor as lazy, calling them takers. When you have grown up with wealth and connections. The world is your oyster. How could you ever know what it is like to be without confidence, food or shelter? How could these people understand the huge mental burden? They can't and most will never even try. Even the self made can find it easy to forget. Like it or not, monetary wealth gives confidence and makes people feel important.

Toxic People Create Toxic Systems

To be healthy, mental health is equally as important as physical health. We have toxic systems because our food, politics, and environment are toxic. So are the people running them. They create these systems on purpose. For example, look at Florida.

The government admitted they created the unemployment website to be as difficult, confusing, and burdensome as possible. "Having studied how [the unemployment system] was internally constructed, I think the goal was for whoever designed, it was, 'Let's put as many kind of pointless roadblocks along the way, so people just say, oh, the hell with it, I'm not going to do that,' " Gov. Ron DeSantis told a Miami CBS affiliate in 2020.

"It was definitely done in a way to lead to the least number of claims being paid out." This is government thinking. The words say they work for us, but they actively work against us using our tax dollars to repress us further. All the while enriching themselves and their corporate donors. Just more proof of the upside-down world we live in.

Assailing us from all sides, dulling and invading our senses, "they" bombard our systems with junk food, chemicals, pills, sugars, and advertisements that tell us it's OK. Treat yourself, give in to that craving, you deserve it.

Very well knowing that all this creates addiction and distraction, dumbing and numbing us down. At the same time they create products of convenience so that we have more time to spend with their burdensome regulations working for them to make them richer.

Complacent, tired, addicted, and worn out humans are easy to manipulate. If we are too busy, slowed down, stressed out from work, bills, life, and our food, then we don't have time to think or question. Never mind attempting to elicit change. It is time to re-prioritize!

CHAPTER NINE

Ingredients

Without great ingredients you will never have great results. This can be said for just about everything. Quality is important. Production, care, weather, soil, preparation, packing, harvesting, picking, netting, catching, killing, foraging, storing, handling, transporting, and processing. Think about the numerous variables and steps that steak, garlic, fish, coffee, banana, chocolate, or kiwi has taken to sit on the shelf for you to eat.

Loss Of Nutrients

Since 1975 there has been a significant loss of nutrient uptake into the food supply. Plants are not getting the same amount of nutrients from the soil as they did forty years ago. It's possible to draw a conclusion as to why.

This loss happens to coincide with the introduction of chemical fertilizers, corporate farms, and pesticides on a massive industrial scale. What is fertilizer after all? Most synthetic fertilizers are a product of the gas and oil industries. Studies have shown that synthetic nitrogen fertilizers lead to reduced microbial content in the soil when compared to organic fertilizers. Because organic fertilizer feeds the soil, while synthetics only feed the plant.

Microorganisms in the soil work with the roots of plants to convert the nutrients and minerals into bioavailable components. Plants then uptake these nutrients through the roots. Healthier soil improves soil structure, nutrient availability and water-holding capacity. Which can reduce the need for watering. Leading to better aeration promoting deeper root growth, and less soil erosion.

It's not a stretch to state that corporate agriculture, lack of cover cropping, high chemical and pesticide usage leads to less microbial diversity in the soil. Resulting in nutrient deficiencies in plants. Creating more need for gas and oil based fertilizers. Is it starting to sound like a familiar story?

In humans nutrient deficiencies directly translate into lower quality of life, more disease, slower thinking and lower IQs. In addition, there is another, more obvious form of destroying food's nutritional content and flavor—early harvesting. The overwhelming majority of today's food has been harvested early. Some foods travel for months. This results in significant losses in nutritional value. Not to mention the negative effects on flavor and texture. Which is unavoidable due to plant respiration, even with refrigeration.

Local And Organic Are The Best Choice

It's a sound cliché, but it's true. As I mentioned already, Chef Dan Barber has proven this. It is a scientific fact. Freshly harvested, local, organic produce will almost always be the most healthy and probably also the best tasting. I say almost because as I discuss later, inputs matter.

Allowing edible produce to remain on the plant until ripening, and eating it shortly after being picked. Is truly the only way to let that ingredient meet its full nutritional and energetic potential. No spin can take away this truth. Most importantly, it's the only way to meet human needs for ideal cognitive and physical function in today's modern society.

For example, a green bell pepper is not ripe. Nor is a green jalapeño pepper. However, they do weigh more and take significantly less time to harvest, when compared to ripe red ones. These singular vegetables are just two examples of the manipulation of food. These peppers are not grown for humans to get the most nutritional value or flavor. Neither are they grown to ripen and eat when ready.

Instead they are grown as a manipulated, commodified unit. Strategically and thoroughly examined. Bred to reap the highest profit, more times than not, by a giant agricultural corporation. The corporation, which by its standard charter must put profits and shareholders first. Does this even qualify as food?

Carbon Dioxide Reduces Nutrient Densities

There's another point to be aware of regarding nutrients in food. Some studies have shown that, as CO_2 levels are increasing, the nutrient densities in plants and vegetables have been decreasing. Specifically, some studies were done with rice—a major source of carbohydrates for a significant portion of the world's population.

Our "food" is barely food at all when it is sprayed with herbicides and fungicides. Add in all the processing, preservatives, early harvesting, and chemical ingredients and it's no wonder that most of what we buy at the supermarket in the United States and call "food" makes us overweight, slow, dour, and sick. Corporate agriculture does not care to remedy this. Profits always come first in this upside-down system. Food is one of our energetic connections to nature. This energy however, has been thoroughly corrupted.

Ingredients Include Medicines

Let us consider that all of the things we ingest are considered ingredients in our diet. We cannot talk about ingredients without talking about medicines with a sober look. It is possible to decipher much of healthcare doesn't heal by solving health problems. At best it's purpose is to mask the problems, usually only temporarily. Probably, much of it is not meant to heal and rather to turn a profit.

There was a time, not so long ago, when advertising drugs on TV was banned in America, but not any more. Every commercial break there are five different ads for legal drugs you can take. Just a mere suggestion to humans. They may have this ailment and this pill will help, is enough to convince people to go to their doctor and ask for the name brand. This is not healthcare, it is suggestive coercion.

Why would there be any reason to advertise pharmaceuticals on TV? This is sick care convincing people, who probably are not in need of this drug. That they may indeed be sick. It is psychological manipulation.

Don't get me wrong. There have been great strides in medicine and there are genuine applications that are beneficial toward helping and healing people and changing their lives for the better. There is also a lot, I'd say the majority, of fluff.

Why bother to consider the root cause of the problem when you can pop some pills and keep acting like everything is normal? Never considering the many chemically derived, added ingredients: preservatives, sugar, corn syrup, maltose, dextrose, sucrose, fructose, caffeine, forever chemicals, pollution in the air, water, our clothes, shampoo, cosmetics, furniture. You can just pop an aspirin, anti-depressant, sleep aid, or rub in a cream. The list of harmful chemicals in everything counts into the hundreds of thousands. Why are humans so trusting that this is OK? Because we don't really get a say?

Why Is Benzene Found In Many Products?

In March 2022 independent testing by a lab called Valisure found that hundreds of personal care products contained benzene. Major name brand shampoos, deodorant, and sunscreens were the worst offenders. Benzene is highly carcinogenic. "Decades" of study shows that there are no safe levels of benzene.

David Light, Valisure's CEO said, "Benzene really shouldn't be there at all. What we are seeing is a fundamental problem in the manufacturing of a lot of consumer products." Yet the FDA allows its use in the production of consumer care products. Where does benzene come from? Do you want to guess? Petroleum of course.

Most people probably don't want to know how harmful their deodorant is. The chemical lobby is huge and has a lot of money. Are we so weak, numb and helpless? Just shouting freedom in anger instead of intelligence? Many will shrug and say, what can I do?

For one you could stop buying deodorant. Shave your armpits. Since, most of the smell comes from bacteria in the hair under your arms anyway. Which brings me to another connection. When I don't drink and eat healthy. I rarely smell and I have not worn deodorant since university. What I noticed is that it's only after I've been drinking, smoking weed or eating a bunch of junk food that I begin to smell and sweat a lot.

Keep Pretending Like Everything Is Fine

So it goes on. Pop an antacid, antibiotic, antidepressant, and pain reliever. Get some chemotherapy. Drink a bottle of wine, vodka, tequila, some beers and whiskey. Keep on doing whatever we want like nothing is happening to our bodies at all. Never wondering why we have these problems. Never asking why we need all these products. Acting like machines.

Humans have become numb and disconnected. Instead of treating the underlying cause, we are just sweeping the problems under the rug where they fester. This, in my opinion, is by design. How could it not be done on purpose?

There is even a political party in America whose politicians are on record stating the quiet part out loud. Saying basically, that the dumber (and number) the masses, the easier they are to control.

Sugar, Processed Foods And Alcohol

I personally don't eat any processed sugars, or processed foods ever. And have lived this way for a long time. Moreover, I stopped drinking alcohol for 6 years. Which really gave me perspective. There are many good reasons to give up drinking alcohol. Besides hangovers, mental health, sleep quality and the dreaded "walk of shame."

A study run by University of Pennsylvania and published in 2022 in Nature Communications found that drinking alcohol actually shrinks your brain. When your gray matter has less volume it leads to "cognitive impairments." Regularly drinking just one drink a day, depending on your age (those who are older suffer more shrinkage), will increase brain aging by one to two years. UPenn professor Gideon Nave stated that the effect is exponential.

Meaning two or three drinks a day accelerated brain aging to more than ten years. In America during the pandemic people drank a lot. According to The International Wines and Spirits Record (IWSR) alcohol consumption in the United States increased by 2% in 2020 to the highest level in 18 years. It's no wonder people started drinking bleach to kill COVID, and began believing in the many ridiculous conspiracy theories.

Alcohol And Sleep

For me personally, alcohol really messes with my sleep and according to the NIH it's not just me. Drinking alcohol to sleep is not as productive as you may think. The NIH says, "Persons who consume alcohol in excessive amounts suffer from poor sleep quality and patients with alcohol use disorders commonly report insomnia." According to the Sleep Foundation "more than 2 drinks for men and more than 1 drink for women will decrease your sleep quality by 39.2%."

I should also mention how important sleep is to your health. Sleep helps your brain and body rebuild itself. Sleep plays a key role in cognitive abilities, cardiovascular, gastrointestinal and immune system functions. It is also very important for mental health, reducing anxiety, depression and rumination. Lack of sleep can also cause hallucinations. While a good night's rest helps maintain focus for longer periods. It also can boost problem solving and athletic abilities. Better sleep correlates with more critical thinking skills, go figure.

Not Sleeping Well Is More Detrimental Than You May Think

While a lack of sleep can cause anxiety, irritability, loss of focus, loss of memory, poor decision making, loss of coordination, poor reasoning, decrease the ability to learn new things and can cause hormonal changes and inflammation. Lack of sleep is also linked to heart disease and diabetes risk. Poor sleep even contributes to weight gain.

Everyone should be taking sleep more seriously if they want to feel good and function at their best performative state. People saying "I will sleep when I am dead" will most likely die sooner, get Alzheimer's or have health issues. Combine brain shrinkage from excess alcohol consumption and poor sleep and you have a recipe for poor health, paranoia, and bad decision making.

This Is Not To Say I am Anti-Fermentation

Since I work in fermentation. I have to admit, I love the concept behind the production of alcoholic beverages. The myriad of unique flavor profiles, the many techniques and styles. Fermented drinks are a part of human civilization. Many are beneficial for your health and contain just a small amount of alcohol. It's the industrialization that's what is concerning.

My point here is that there's a time and place for everything, in moderation. In the United States there are also many chemical additives in most commercial beers, wines and liquors. Trusting major alcohol companies to do what's right for your health is never a good idea.

I personally enjoy the flavor of naturally made, sugar free champagne, sulfite free natural wine and mezcal. But almost always, drinking alcohol will make me feel depressed and lazy for the next day or two, after even just one drink. These are both feelings I don't like. They are also feelings, that when millions of people combined are feeling them, contribute to a lack of motivation to change the paradigm.

I hate to admit it but alcoholism is a huge part of the problem humanity faces. I'd go so far as to say it's probably a major factor in the reason why America is the way it is right now. According to the 2019 National Survey on Drug Use and Health 59% of men and 51% of women 18 and older reported drinking alcohol in the past month. Many people drink to cope, but the unintended consequences are too real.

I'm Gonna Say It (Don't Laugh) I Get High On Life

I personally get my high these days from mediation and exercise. They do really make you feel great when combined with a healthy diet. In the past, I pushed myself to the extreme. Drinking as we referred to it, at a competitive level. Simultaneously, the whole time smoking weed.

After I quit everything for many years and reset my reality. I realized that I can still drink or smoke occasionally. Because now I am totally in control. I am prepared for the mental and physical consequences. And you notice them, and you remember them. And you don't like them.

Still to this day the recognition and understanding of myself gives me the answer that being clean is infinitely more enjoyable and opportune. Taking an hour a day just for yourself is all you need. Thirty minutes of mediation and 10-20 minutes of stretching and exercise does wonders.

Obviously, I am strict when it comes to food. Only eating organically grown food. I am fortunate we have a farmers market all year long in Ojai and in France the whole system is much better than in the states.

Eating this way does make it difficult to eat out at many restaurants. But I find that I feel much healthier than I ever have before.

The Truth About Most Restaurants

I happened to work in the restaurant industry during my high school and university years. Gaining a good understanding of how things work in the industry. You may be surprised how much of a restaurant's food comes from major corporate distributors, and even cans. Especially chain and franchise restaurants. Eating out at one of these is pretty much the same as eating TV dinners. The majority of restaurants are buying the cheapest bulk food they can and dressing it up. Profits are often the first consideration in the restaurant business, because profit margins are usually very thin.

Who doesn't like it when someone else cooks and does the dishes? Cooking probably isn't fun for most people. I personally don't like to cook. So it's understandable, but eating out regularly, for the most part, can pose a health risk if you're not extremely critical of the establishment.

My Personal Diet

Ninety-eight percent of my diet is fiber rich, and includes veggies, greens, nuts, grains, and fruits. I eat duck eggs (when possible), which are higher in protein and nutrients. I always make sure to maximize nutrition by seeking out specific foods with the highest nutrient densities, fiber, vitamins and minerals. Every single morning I eat organic plain oatmeal with a full cup of organic frozen (or fresh when available) blueberries or raisins. When I'm traveling I pack oatmeal with raisins.

Since I started this habit it has really improved my brain function. I can actually feel it. Harvard nutritional psychiatrist Uma Naidoo says blueberries are her number one brain food. Packed with flavonoids, antioxidants, fiber and folate. Blueberries can boost your mood, ward off dementia, lower inflammation in your gut and brain, and improve gut health.

Nothing Is Easy, But If You Want To, You Can Do Anything

I admit that converting to this way of living was not easy. However, with practice you will master it. For me it is not only a habit now, but also has become easy. Once you decipher what is available, what you like and the different ways to prepare said ingredients, it all becomes second nature. No different than building any habit really.

Living this way, I have been able to truly see the world for what it is, and to think clearly. One super side effect is that my sense of smell became incredibly strong. The difference in how I feel is significant when compared to the way I lived before. No more "food coma," not ever. I always have lots of energy and I sleep very well and feel rested when I wake up.

You can do this too. The point is to be able to be objective so you will be able to realize how significantly the ingredients in your diet affect your life, decision making and health. But to find this objectivity you have to cut out everything that is not the most basic of foods. For a significant period of time. It will take more than a year to detox a lifetime of toxins. And you will most likely suffer withdrawals and have healing crises.

The FDA And Corporations Will Not Protect Your Health

You alone have to be the protector of your health. No one should expect food purveyors, the government or the FDA to take your best interests into consideration.

We cannot expect those in power to protect your health. These same people who, for the most part, are not mentally or physically healthy. Are there to uphold the status quo.

Would you let a drunk hold the keys to the liquor cabinet or drive your car? Why do we trust corrupt and incompetent people to steer the ship while they themselves are in cahoots with the pirates? Proper ship captains go through rigorous testing and have to maintain sobriety when they are on duty.

Why shouldn't this apply to our politicians and business leaders? Almost no one is operating at 100% of their full cognitive potential and they are definitely operating with only one or two things in mind, profits and power.

Power Does Not Care About Health

During the pandemic, for example, governments will regulate people to stay locked at home. Ordering convenience food and alcohol to cope. Yet, the same governments will never mandate big agriculture, big pharma, and chemical corporations remove the toxins from our water and food supplies. To protect long term health. Which is worse? If everyone were healthier, they most likely would be a lot less afraid because they know they have a strong immune system and are thinking more clearly, acting less out of a state of fear.

Don't you want to know what "meds" your politicians are taking? How about how much they drink? You should want to know. Considering how pharmaceuticals and alcohol affects brain function. There have been many American presidents and congressmen who have been known to be drinkers. Shouldn't these people be operating at their best mental capacity to run the country?

An airline pilot or ship captain will be fired if they drink on the job. They are only responsible for a few hundred lives at a time. Politicians manage hundreds of millions of lives every day. Many of these same politicians want to impose drug tests on poor people in need of food stamps, unemployment and government assistance. But they will never regulate themselves. Especially, if they are getting donations to take a side.

The Number Of People Popping Pills Daily Is Staggering

I am not talking about antibiotics. In 2021, approximately 55% of Americans were taking pharmaceuticals, daily. Let me say it another way. More than half of America takes prescription drugs every day. These drugs alter thinking, personalities, energetic signatures and change the behaviors of the people taking them. It's not a stretch to say that America is in this situation because no one can think clearly.

If you are on an antidepressant, you certainly don't have the will power to make an effort to take a stand. I have taken an antidepressant one time in my life. One half of a Paxil. It made me so OK with everything I was numb. You could tell me you shoot puppies. I would have just smiled and said, "that's cool."

Numb Is Complacent

Here we are with more than half the country, including children, getting numb. Just pop some aspirin, a digestive aid, a muscle relaxant, something to keep you awake, something to make you focus or an antidepressant. Everything will be fine and stay the same. Of course, when you live in the upside-down world. How could it be anything other than purposefully designed this way?

Why do you think the government decided to let pharmaceutical companies advertise on TV again? These people know that our environments are messing up our bodies and brains so they can keep making drugs to "fix" us.

A Handful Of Corporations Control The Food Supply

The Guardian with Food and Water Watch did a joint investigation To show how choice is actually not what it seems for Americans. They found that almost 80% of everyday grocery items are produced by only a handful of companies; 93% of sodas are owned by three companies; only three companies dominate 73% of cereals. And more than 80% of beef and 70% of pork processing is run by four giant conglomerates. This is one reason it is so important to support local and organic. We have to vote for the world we want with the money we spend.

In the 1970s, under President Nixon, the government literally instituted a war on food. A full 95% of American grain reserves became under the control of just six companies. Henry Kissinger famously said, "Control food and you control the people." Traditional Agriculture has been systematically replaced by Big Agriculture.

The US government has essentially engineered these controlling strategies for over 50 years now, putting the entire world under its thumb. A docile, compliant population is much easier to control. Humans have to stop, think, and listen. But can't stop, think, and listen because food and society has been corrupted so thoroughly. Precisely to keep us from stopping, thinking, and listening to ourselves. To stop us from taking action.

Chemicals In Alcohol

It is not just chemicals in our food. It's beverages and beer too. Anheuser-Busch alone owns more than 600 beer brands. You may not even be aware. There are over one thousand chemicals approved as additives for the alcohol industry. The craziest part? Alcohol companies are not required to list any ingredients on the label.

So much booze has corn syrup and many other chemicals in it. Yet, you will never even know under the current system of labeling, even if you ask. Add some chemicals and a few pills. Who knows how the combined effects will alter your thoughts, perceptions, and behaviors.

Chemical Usage Is Growing Exponentially

How about pesticides and herbicides? Does anyone actually believe that we can continue putting these chemicals on crops and food without them contaminating the environment or our ingredients and bodies? Of course not. But it keeps happening.

Researchers at George Washington University examined urine samples from just over 14,000 people, ages six and older. They were looking for exposure to a herbicide called 2, 4-D. They found that one in three Americans have detectable levels of 2, 4-D in their bodies. If you are familiar with Agent Orange, used in the Vietnam war, one of the ingredients is 2, 4-D.

This herbicide is linked to leukemia in children, birth defects, reproductive problems, cancer, and hormonal imbalances. Wonder why you have an acne outbreak, are feeling depressed or hormonally imbalanced? Maybe it's from all the 2, 4-D you have been exposed to (and it's not just 2, 4-D that has these effects).

2, 4-D has been shown to disrupt the endocrine system which controls growth, reproduction, moods, and our metabolism. In an interesting twist, more white people were shown to have been exposed to 2, 4-D than black people.

Roughly 600 products in America contain 2, 4-D which can be ingested through the skin, nose, and mouth. In the past decade, use of 2, 4-D has risen over 65%, and the researchers predict that with the use of genetically modified crops. Usage of 2, 4-D will unfortunately continue to rise as well.

Vote For Change With Buying And Actions

How can humans take back control of their health, ingredients, and the environment? We can do this, not only by demanding bans on these types of chemicals, but through a concerted effort to educate ourselves as well. Insisting on only purchasing organic produce and refusing to buy conventional types of products. The only way to make a product obsolete is to eliminate the market for it. Vote with your money.

Some will say, but organic costs more. I think maybe this is a short sighted argument. What you save in the short term ends up being 10,000 times or more back into the pockets of the healthcare system in the long term.

The white picket fence and weed free, green lawn. Who sold these ideas to us in the first place? Corporate messaging and homeowners associations who wanted to force everyone into conformity.

If we rethink the idea of a weed free suburban green lawn. Making our yards into a natural environment and vegetable garden instead. We will help to refute the idea of manufactured perfection, while producing our own food and eliminating the need for weed killers (2, 4-D).

Sure it's easier to just spray something than actually removing the weeds ourselves. But it's a lot less gratifying than growing our own food and supporting our health, the natural environment, bees, birds, butterflies, and all living things. Gardens grow life!

Water Is Tainted Everywhere On The Planet

Water is an essential ingredient in everything. It is the most consumed beverage on Earth. It is also essential for our day to day survival. However, our waterways are polluted with sex changing hormones, pharmaceuticals and many other pollutants. It's not that there aren't many studies out there that show the truth of this. It's just that nothing is being done to stop it.

Researchers at Florida International University's Coastal Fisheries Research Lab identified 58 different pharmaceuticals in bonefish off the coast of South Florida, Caribbean, Bahamas, Puerto Rico, Mexico and Belize. Bonefish are a multi-billion dollar sport fishing industry. The average drug concoction per fish was seven pharmaceuticals, yet some fish had as many at sixteen different pharmaceuticals in the flesh.

The researchers also found similar contaminants in crabs, shrimp, water and sediment. You may be asking yourself, "how did these drugs get into the sea water in the first place?" The lead researcher for the study, Dr. Jennifer Rehage says, "conventional wastewater treatment in Florida and other parts of the United States does not remove pharmaceuticals. It's in our drinking water. We also have it in our fish that we consume."

It's true, there are no regulations governing disposal of pharmaceuticals. "So, they're not considered a contaminant." Interesting take the government has on this situation. A doctor has to prescribe these drugs found in fish; Clorpromazine (antipsychotic), Flupentixol (antipsychotic), Codeine (opioid), Oxazepam (antidepressant), Paroxetine (antidepressant), Dicycloverine (stomach medication for IBS), Clotrimazol (antifungal cream) and Valium (muscle relaxant / anxiety medication). But, once these chemicals are in the water (and fish). There's nothing anyone can do about it right?

So the government's position on this is; too bad if you don't want to take pharmaceuticals. What's a little fungal cream and a dash of antipsychotic with your tap water and grilled fish plate gonna hurt? This type of thing makes me outraged. I don't consent to putting these drugs in my body. You have to ask, are there any clean foods left? Are there any places that are not contaminated? It would seem that there are not.

Sex Changes In Fish And Frogs

We can see the hormonal effects in the species living within contaminated waterways. Scientists from the U.S. Fish and Wildlife Service and the U.S. Geological Survey undertook studies in 19 national wildlife areas in the Northeast United States. They found that 60-100% of male smallmouth bass are intersex.

In Vermont, at the Missisquoi National Wildlife Refuge—which happens to be one of the most productive and pristine wetland ecosystems in the Northeast—about 85% of male smallmouth bass are intersex. In this case meaning they are growing female egg sacs in their testes. Feminized male fish have been found in 37 species all over the world.

This is also prevalent in frogs which are turning from males into females, something not known to happen naturally in amphibians. One culprit is a pesticide known as atrazine which affects testosterone production.

Even when you go fishing in the most pristine wetlands and think you are catching a clean 'natural' fish, when you eat it you are consuming atrazine or pharmaceuticals. This is the new "natural" world we live in.

How Do These Chemicals Affect Human Development?

This information made me stop and consider. All over the Earth there are strong anti LGBTQ stances taking place. From citizens, organizations and religious groups to governments. Do any of these anti LGBTQ people stop to question how this increase in people identifying as gay is happening?

It's very possible, the increase in people identifying as LGBTQ has happened because of the thousands of hormone and endocrine disrupting chemicals in the environment. Which people have been consuming since birth.

In a Gallup Poll 15.9% of Gen Z (those born in the late 1990s to early 2000s) identified as LGBTQ. I don't want this to be taken out of context here. I completely support the LGBTQ community and believe that everyone is equal and should be treated as so.

My point here, does anyone consider that maybe the environment we live in could be affecting people's bodies? If fish and frogs are changing sex due to contaminated water, you can't deny the possibility.

Don't Think Just Divide

Thinking and troubleshooting our problems seems to be a far off concept for politicians. I personally fear humans can't and don't think anymore. It's easier to blame and use the LGBTQ community as a cudgel to divide and tribalize, caught up in the culture wars! It's a consistent theme, blame someone else.

What is at issue with the state of the human mind? It is so very toxic and broken. Not only are we dumbing down our population with chemicals and less nutrient dense food. But also with the air we breathe.

Duke University and Florida State University published a peer reviewed study in University Proceedings of the National Academy of Sciences in early 2022. They found that people born from the 1940s through to the 1980s, approximately 170 million people, lost as much as seven IQ points from the use of leaded gasoline. Simply due to breathing exhaust fumes.

More Profits

Why did the gasoline companies put lead in the gasoline in the first place? If I say "more profits," will you be shocked? Simply put, in order for a combustion engine to have a more consistent performance they needed to improve the octane rating. Today's average is 87-93 octane. But back in the 1930s and 1940s the octane rating was only 40-60.

The oil companies had a choice. Here comes a constant theme. Further refine the gasoline so it had a higher octane rating, or find an additive. I will leave you to guess which was cheaper. That additive is called tetraethyl-lead. "Childhood lead exposure is not just here and now. It's going to impact your lifelong health," said Abheet Solomon, a senior program manager at the United Nations Children's Fund.

Bruce Lanphear, a health sciences professor at Simon Fraser University in Vancouver said "The more tragic part is that we keep making the same ... mistakes again," Lanphear said. "First it was lead, then it was air pollution. ... Now it's PFAS chemicals and phthalates (chemicals used to make plastics more durable). And it keeps going on and on. And we can't stop long enough to ask ourselves should we be regulating chemicals differently."

As long as the government puts profits before people. These same systems will give priority to money, power, division, and control over human health, leaving a clean environment and healthy ingredients to come last. This must be changed. This upside-down world must be turned right-side up.

CHAPTER TEN

Sugar

Thanks to hundreds of years of large scale production, sugar is the world's most energetically corrupt, legal addictive substance. The history of sugar is quite a long story. There are many books that detail this history in great lengths.

I couldn't write this book without dedicating a chapter to sugar. The energetic negativity and full frontal impact it has on society, the exploitation of the workers, the control the sugar lobby has over the government—it's just incredible. I want to briefly detail some of the highlights to give some historical perspective and background.

History Of Sugar

Sugar has been cultivated for about 10,000 years, supposedly starting in New Guinea. Its recipes go back as far as 2,500 years, spanning the Roman times to the British and American colonies. Sugar interests controlled the British parliament. Sugar funded the British empire and navy. A British tax on sugar helped fuel the fire of the revolutionary activities of the American colonies.

Over 11 Million people were enslaved to harvest and cultivate sugar. Mostly these people were stolen from Africa. Enslaved people were sent to the Caribbean and Southern United States to work on plantations. Raw sugar cane would be harvested by hand and needed to be boiled down to crystals and molasses immediately. Because cane juice ferments very quickly, the labor and speed necessary was backbreaking.

The raw product would then be shipped to the new world to process. New York City was a major sugar refining center from colonial times until recently. When they turned the Domino Sugar factory in Williamsburg, Brooklyn into condos. In the 19th century, behind the Trinity church in downtown Manhattan, there used to be a five story warehouse full of sugar stretching all the way to the East River.

The Sweetest And Most Addictive Substance Known To Man

Cane sugar is the sweetest natural substance known to mankind. It activates each of our ten thousand receptors on our taste buds. It also happens to be more addictive than cocaine. There are stories of rats becoming so addicted to sugar they would not eat anything else and would die from starvation if sugar was not available.

The waste product of sugar production is molasses. The entire rum industry was spawned solely to make use of the molasses. This industry created countless problems and more slavery. I won't even detail the horrors here. There's an entire other story about slaves, rum, and alcoholism.

Originally Sugar Was Only Available To The Wealthy

Just like tea, originally sugar was very expensive and only available to the wealthy. The upper classes would have parties and make sugar sculptures to demonstrate their wealth and power. Not only that, they also made cups and saucers out of sugar as well. When tea service was done, guests would eat the cups and saucers or take the remainder home with them.

One author on sugar pondered why Renaissance paintings never depicted any one smiling. His answer, likely because everyone's teeth were rotten from eating sugar. In the 18th and 19th centuries with the introduction of tea and coffee and some technological advances in harvesting, sugar started to become more widely available for the masses. This spawned the candy industry.

Sugar Is Big Money

Fast forward to the present day. Sugar production in America is around nine million tons annually. The sugar industry receives approximately $3-4 billion in subsidies each year. Americans on average consume in excess of forty pounds of sugar in the form of sucrose. When adding in all forms of sweeteners, the total per person is over seventy pounds per year. The sugar crop in Louisiana alone generates about $3 billion in revenue each year.

Florida is the largest production region in the US with over 200,000 acres. Only two companies account for the majority of the sugar production in Florida. This is because the American Sugar Program subsidizes prices by buying any excess, limiting the amount of production stateside and enforcing quotas on imports. American taxpayers are contributing to the enormous wealth of only a handful of major corporations and one family in particular. This family's history of exploitation and political donating is very long.

A Lot Of Political Donations And Lobbying

The sugar industry only employs a few thousand workers. The industry however, spends enormous sums of money hiring lobbyists. The sugar industry accounts for roughly 2% of American crops by value in the United States. Yet, sugar companies account for nearly 30% of campaign contributions by crop producing companies.

It's a simple and very profitable system really: make campaign contributions to politicians using taxpayer subsidies to ensure that the same subsidies keep flowing. This system benefits only a few people at the expense of the environment, workers, and taxpayers. Not to mention the cost to human health.

How Sugar Plantations Affect The Environment In Florida

In Florida most of the sugarcane is grown just South of Lake Okeechobee. In the 1950s, two thousand miles of levees and canals were created in a project called the Everglades Agricultural Area. This project turned what was once marshland into an agricultural area.

This area also happened to be the perfect spot to grow sugar cane. Unfortunately, these canals disrupted the flow of fresh water into the Florida bay. Which in turn disrupted the living environment and salinity levels in the bay. After many decades the state of Florida came up with a solution.

This solution included not renewing a lease for the biggest sugar conglomerate in the world. This would deprive this company of 10% of the land solely in the Everglades Agricultural Area. A fraction of their crop globally.

Surely, for the sake of the environment and benefit for the people of Florida. One of the biggest sugar companies in the world, funded by taxpayer subsidies, could do the right thing. But no, that solution was blocked, and the lease was renewed last minute by the local water board.

The water board just so happens to be a political organization. Yet, clearly doesn't work for Florida residents' best interests. When only greed, money, and power are allowed to dictate environmental policy, nothing good will come for the many at the expense of the few.

The Negative Energy Associated With Sugar Is Unimaginable

There are so many egregious examples throughout history of bad behavior associated with the sugar industry. One cannot even fathom the negative energy associated with it. For example, just as the tobacco companies and oil companies have done, sugar companies in the 1960s paid Harvard scientists to produce research that downplayed the connection between sugar and heart disease. Instead laying the blame on saturated fat.

Once a crop of exploitation, always a crop of exploitation. Until this very day it is said that the sugar mills and producers let some minorities own land and supply crops specifically for the purpose of getting large government loans.

Per the NY Times, Eddie Lewis III stated, "You need a few minorities in there, because these mills survive off having minorities involved with the mill to get these huge government loans." Eddie Lewis III is a former Morgan Stanley financial advisor who left his banking career to become a fifth generation farmer. He is one of the few Black individuals to own a sugar farm. The American Sugar Cane League is said to highlight (exploit) him since he is one of only a handful of Black farm owners in Louisiana.

To this day in Louisiana there are still 'slaves' harvesting sugar. Although, they call them prisoners now. The Angola maximum security prison—the largest prison by landmass—also happens to be a sugar plantation.

The Many Names Of Sugar

Sugar feeds diabetes, obesity, and cancer. The words "sugar free" on a product's packaging does not always mean the product is sweetener free. Sugars and sweeteners in the United States are listed under fifty-six different names. Many are named from the source of the sweetener.

However, many people would not be able to identify these names as sugar unless you took the time to learn. Dextrose, galactose, maltose, maltodextrin, ethyl maltol, golden syrup, and dextrin, to name a few of the obscure derivatives. There are fifteen names legally used to refer to sugar directly. The other forty-one are considered sugar substitutes or sweeteners.

These hidden, and not so hidden sugars are in more than two thirds of barcoded products. This doesn't account for the ones that are not barcoded. Like fast food french fries. Sugar or corn syrup are often the first and second ingredients in many products. Many times it is both! Do you need to ask why?

Why Every Company Fills Products With The Most Addictive Substance On Earth

Companies may obfuscate by saying it acts as a preservative. Or that sugar helps retain water, or makes bread fluffier. Or that sugar brings out the flavor. These are all true. However, the whole truth I will repeat again. Sugar is one of, if not the most addictive substance on Earth.

If you are a company and want the customer to keep buying a product what do you do? Put the most addictive, legal substance on Earth in it. Why do you think Coca Cola used to have cocaine in it? Now instead they use something even better, 39 grams of sugar (per 12oz can) to be exact. Or in the "sugar free" and "diet" versions they use some derivatives.

Sugar Is In Everything

I stopped eating cane sugar and processed sugars in 2015. The only sugars I consume now are natural fruit sugars, when I eat fruit. I don't even eat honey anymore unless I am able to watch it harvested from the hive and question the producer.

The vast majority of honey is adulterated and has sweeteners, antibiotics and corn syrup in it. I don't mean to say honey has antibiotic properties. Literally, the bees are fed a sugar syrup solution with antibiotics, in the hive to help keep them healthy. Unfortunately, this translates into contaminated honey.

In my desire to become truly free and healthy, I had to cut out sugar. Cutting out sugar entirely was one of the most difficult tasks I have ever undertaken. It is added to everything; (American) pizza dough, pasta sauce, sushi rice, red and white wines, beer, hard liquor, french fries, bread, ketchup, applesauce, salad dressings, processed meats, cereals and granola, TV dinners, to the most obscure things you would never even think of.

Even if the label says "sugar free" it is most probably not sweetener free. Almost every item in the supermarket contains sugar, corn syrup or one of the derivatives. Many times it is a combination. Even pet food has sugar in it. Over the years I became an expert at finding this hidden drug.

Sugar Has Many Detrimental Effects To Your Health

You are probably saying to yourself, "This guy is nuts!" Maybe I am. Did you know? Among many other detrimental effects, sugar feeds tumors and cancer cells. This is called the 'Warburg Effect,' named after Dr. Otto Warburg, who won the Nobel Prize in 1931.

He figured out, wait for it… that cancer feeds itself by fermenting sugar. Remember what I said earlier about Auto Brewery Syndrome and the potential for corn syrup to ferment in your gut? Not only that, this process alters your genes by epigenetic expression.

Of course I cannot forget to mention diabetes, addiction, serotonin deficiency and obesity. The trigger for me to cut out sugar was my father's death. He died of stomach cancer which had spread into his intestines.

My Fathers Death Made Me Start Researching

My father was a very healthy, fit man. His body fat was maybe only 2% when he became sick. He was very active and exercised regularly. He was still incredibly muscular and athletic at 65. Which made me wonder what happened.

He loved processed meats, processed cakes, canned soda, and sweet tea. Sandwiches, potato rolls, hot dogs, and TV dinners. As he would say it. He was a red blooded, gun loving, meat and potatoes, Republican voting, Fox News watching American.

I thought how would someone who appeared so healthy on the outside get stomach and intestinal cancer? So I started to look into his diet. Everything he ate contained chemicals and sugar. The chemicals cause cancer and the sugar works like steroids for it.

His diet was filled daily by processed foods with sugar, nitrites and nitrates. He died in 2015. Later that year, the World Health Organization classified all processed meats as a carcinogen and cause of stomach cancer. Due to the nitrites and nitrates contained within them.

My Entire Family Died From Cancer And Disease

My mother was diagnosed with Alzheimers in 2002 and lived with this condition for 21 more years. My grandmother died with dementia. She would go for walks and get lost. Family would have to go look for her. Both my grandfathers had multiple cancers, heart attacks, and strokes. They all died from cancer. So I looked at their diets too. What did I find? Meat and potatoes, alcoholism, lack of exercise.

Growing up Polish, potatoes were always on the menu. Conventionally grown potatoes are one of what is called the "dirty dozen." These are the most heavily sprayed foods. Potatoes are not only coated in pesticides but fungicides as well. At fast food restaurants they add sugar to the mix. Some even add bleach to this toxic cocktail.

Take a "conventional" potato and a traditionally grown "organic" potato. Side by side, leave them and wait. Watch how fast buds will spout on the "organic" one. Conventional potatoes are sprayed after harvesting so that they don't sprout those buds.

This increases their shelf life at the expense of decreasing the life expectancy of the person consuming them. My grandparents and my mother all also happened to love sweets. Cancer causing chemicals, plus sugar, equals death in my family. I'm sure it's not just my family.

After I cut out sugar from my diet. My brain function and energy levels normalized, and got my taste buds back. I realized my taste buds had been burnt out. Because sugar activates every single receptor on your tongue. Things that were naturally sour, never tasted as sour as they had before. I started to detect the actual flavor of food. Just regular old unseasoned food suddenly became appealing and flavorful again. This is one of the greatest benefits for me.

Sure, I miss creme brûlée and baklava. However, I have to tell you that I feel absolutely fantastic! You can too and you don't have to go as far as I did. But you have to go far enough to get clean first.

CHAPTER ELEVEN

Upside Down

Pay the fee, get vested.
Mind the guardrails, pop
goes the unicorn.
Formulaic, on repeat.
Courage, ethical speak,
we may not seek.
For within the legal limits,
must it be fine, must it be usual,
to fall within the lines,
of those who have built us
upside-down.

The Value Of A Human Life

Various US government agencies value each American life in the realm of $8-10 million USD. These agencies use a formula where a VSL is calculated. VSL stands for Value of a Statistical Life. When these agencies want to implement a new regulation. They are calculating whether the benefits will outweigh the costs.

It's not surprising, but I bet most people don't have much idea how the government operates internally. If it were common knowledge how statisticians and economists build countries, economies, and budgets.

The revelation would find that every human life has a monetary value. Like livestock, humans are no differently counted than cattle. Citizens are merely a means to an end.

The Politicians Are Supposed to Work For the Citizens

Who is the government anyway? The wording says the politicians work for us and we hire them with votes of confidence. If everyday citizens were to lie, cheat, steal, and act the way politicians do in their jobs. Surely they will be fired or worse, arrested.

Politicians sure seem to act like it is the citizens who owe them. Doing as they wish with tax dollars. It is time citizens remind the politicians they owe us. Our tax dollars pay their salaries. Those are our tax dollars they spend on pet projects to enrich their donors.

Politicians Are Opposite People

Politicians are what I call opposite people. Opposite people project their greatest faults and weaknesses as strengths. They spin and obfuscate everything. Using what is termed political speech to get away with the most egregious of lies.

Most of the time whatever blame they lay on the other is the very thing they are guilty of doing themselves. I find this is especially true with conservative politicians. And it is just so blatantly obvious. Yet, everyday right in front of our faces citizens let them get away with it.

Governing Only To Maintain Power

When the government goes about "governing" us they will say the citizens and the constitution gave them this mandate. I want to ask, who gave them this power in the first place? Who said they should be able to lie, cheat, steal, connive, and divide with impunity? All just to maintain power. They did, since they are the ones that make the laws.

Politicos will argue that it's protected political speech when they lie. It's how business is done when corporations and donors give them money and they make rules and laws that are favorable to their donors. It is all legal, baby, they are just playing by the rules. The rules they made for themselves.

Rules For Thee, Not For Me

When did citizens give up our sovereign right as humans to live freely and express ourselves (outside the very tight guardrails set for us as a society)? There are so many laws in America that every person, every day breaks more than one law. It is no wonder that America is the world's leading jailer. With 5% of the world's population we have 25% of the world's prisoners. More than China!

This is an insane but accurate statistic. With so many stupid laws there is always a way to wield power over citizens and enemies. No point to even mention how the enforcers abuse these laws. I won't even get into the statistics of arrests. Black and brown people obviously suffer disproportionately. If you don't know already, just look at the statistics.

When did citizens become corporate and government assets? Wage and debt slaves? To be placed in prison at any moment of the "authorities" choosing. Based solely on the words of a police officer. Don't citizens always have to prove everything? Our words alone are never considered proof enough.

Why Is There Government Anyway?

Sure, in the ideal sense, the government helps to solve society's ills by creating safety, building highways, bridges, sewers, waterways, et cetera.

In a right-side up world, the government would be a fair, mediating, and protecting entity that does improve the quality of its citizens' lives without micromanaging, imprisoning, misleading or meddling. They would treat citizens with care and protect them from harm. They would trust their citizens and help them flourish, thrive, and be their best selves.

Isn't safety the number one reason the government always gives us as a reason for the government? Societal safety, health safety, and protection is a reason the government comes to be. The concept of government isn't all bad. So it must be the people who operate it that have corrupted it. It is exactly this perversion that has brought us to the point we're at today.

The Government Is One Giant Corporation

When a city comes into being they say it's been "incorporated." The government and all its trade deals and so on are no different than a giant parent corporation or holding company. It's one gigantic corporation seeking endless profit and GDP. Year after year GDP must be ever expanding.

Through taxes, the government gets a cut from all the other corporations and the products under its umbrella. At least from some corporations, anyway. The really big corporations don't even bother to pay taxes. The government pays them our taxes in the form of subsidies. Plus, these companies lobby enough to make the loopholes just big enough for them to slip right through.

Profit Producing Assets

The way the government is presently structured. Citizens are collectively a means to an end. Citizens producing profits, worker debt slaves, living in a consumption based society, consuming massive amounts of resources. It all comes at a cost. That's why America is known as one of the most over-worked nations in the world. With a very small amount of paid medical leave to boot. The US is great at managing their citizens' productivity!

In America, it would seem, citizens live to work. Whereas in France, they say, the French work to live. In America, assets must be maintained to minimize depreciation. Citizens must be tamed, modeled, guided, and trained. Used to the most efficient levels at every turn. Replete with advertising to tell us it's OK, trade yourself for money. Promptly spending that money and giving it right back to the top 1%. This way they get your taxes and your pay.

Pimps And Hoes

Our food is spiked with chemicals, hormones, salt, fat, sugar, and bacteria. Like a pimp has his hoes on smack, the corporations have you hooked. Don't forget about organizations like ALEC (American Legislative Exchange Council) helping to fix the guardrails of our society. There are many other "think tanks" as well, like the Heritage Foundation. ALEC just happens to be one of the most notorious.

ALEC writes model legislation and laws which it lobbies the government to enact on behalf of big business. Does this seem self-serving and corrupt to you? It should, because it is. Yet, it's totally legal corruption. How could it be illegal? That's the nature of big business. They are the ones who help make the laws to benefit themselves.

The Upside-Down World At It's Finest

Put on a suit and tie and take on the role. Place yourself in the other side's shoes. This is the first step to any business negotiation. What is being hidden and why? For an example, why do you think the USDA Organic label came to be? This is just my opinion, but I bet it's not the reason many think.

The absurdity of this speaks volumes. This labeling structure exists solely to charge farms a fee to label organically (without chemical fertilizers or pesticides) grown food. The fees are not cheap either, and they have to be paid yearly. This is incredibly backward. Think about this.

A farm using traditional agricultural practices—farming practices that humans have been using for thousands of years—has to pay a fee to distinguish the products they sell from the farms that are using chemicals.

Instead of the chemically produced products paying fees be regulated and to distinguish themselves from organic products. These are the same chemicals that have been shown to harm the balance of life on Earth, cause cancer and hormonal imbalances amongst numerous other problems.

Big Agriculture is killing off important bacteria in the soils, polluting waterways and causing sex changes in fish frogs, and probably humans. While organic farms are the ones that have to pay fees to separate their produce from the massive, subsidized, corporate agricultural complex. A complex that receives billions of dollars in subsidies from the government every year.

Let me say it another way. The organic farms have to help subsidize the giant, corporate ones. This is the upside-down world we live in. We must right ourselves to see the madness clearly. Situations like this ALEC would support, and probably did. This is the kind of model legislation ALEC would write and hand to the politicians. Who will, more times than not, literally copy and paste it into law. This is the truth about how many laws are made, not an opinion.

Backward Sense Trumps Common Sense

Common sense would dictate that genetically modified foods, grown with chemical fertilizers, additives, and pesticides. Should be clearly marked with some sort of label. This would make more sense than adding bureaucracy, cost, and difficulty to those farming naturally. Farms that are mostly struggling to get by. Farms that don't rely on government subsidies.

The obvious purpose is to create barriers to entry and stifle competition. There is also another purpose: the land grab. Small farms are going extinct in America. The argument the government will give its citizens for the land grab. They have to make sure these farms are truly using organic practices. This argument only makes sense in an upside-down world.

Flip It Right Side Up

If we flip it right-side up, the farms using chemicals will have to be inspected and pay fees every season. Inspectors would come and check the chemicals in use to ensure they are safe and not polluting the waterways, or contaminating the produce, or harming the workers. These fees would also be used to subsidize the smaller organic farms.

Since organic farms are not using chemicals, the inspection process would be much easier. It would also almost certainly stimulate more organic farms into existence. In the right-side up world, produce that is not grown organically or naturally would be labeled accordingly. It would state that these products had been grown with the use of chemicals, fertilizers, herbicides, and fungicides. Like a pack of cigarettes there would be a warning label.

Think of the humble potato. Does it say anywhere on the packaging that these 'conventionally' grown potatoes are sprayed with fungicide? Of course it does not. Instead of adding bureaucracy and cost to farmers using chemical fertilizers. The government adds it to those farmers who are farming in a way that humans have farmed for thousands of years. Does this sound right-side up to you?

The Scale Is Massive

Since these corporate "conventional" chemical farms are operating at such a massive scale. Not to mention that chemical fertilizers make the produce much larger and grow faster. These chemical farms could surely afford the fees to be regulated properly.

Henry Kissinger was right. Control the food supply and you control everything. Big Agriculture has more money to lobby what's in their best interests. More money to donate to politicians. Not to mention the billions in subsidies they receive. Which they turn around and use to rig the game to their advantage. They will never lobby what's in the citizens best interest.

Citizen Tax Dollars Subsidize Harm to The Environment

The small local farms. More often than not are just trying to get by. In the upside-down world we live in. Your tax dollars are subsidizing the very chemicals and companies that are exerting control over us, the environment and our health. You should be outraged. We are paying them to essentially poison us and the Earth. It could not be more backwards.

I have to tell you the industry argument for not labeling chemically grown foods. This is not my opinion. What's the industry argument for not labeling "conventional" food as potentially toxic? Don't scare the customer. Literally, that's the argument. Doesn't this scare you? What is in your food? Seriously, you don't know. But if you want to live and think healthy, then we must turn our world right-side up.

More about subsidies. According to a report by the IMF (International Monetary Fund) the global fossil fuel industry benefits from subsidies at a rate of $11 million per minute. This totaled about $5.9 Trillion in 2020.

Further, the researchers state that ending these subsidies would prevent almost one million deaths per year from polluted air and raise trillions of dollars for governments. "There would be enormous benefits from reform, so there's an enormous amount at stake," said Ian Parry, the lead author of the IMF report.

"Some countries are reluctant to raise energy prices because they think it will harm the poor. But holding down fossil fuel prices is a highly inefficient way to help the poor, because most of the benefits accrue to wealthier households. It would be better to target resources towards helping poor and vulnerable people directly." Taxpayers are subsidizing the wealthiest companies on the planet to continue destroying the planet. While making the already super rich, richer.

It is not only oil, sugar, and agricultural companies, but also beef production, deforestation, groundwater pumping, and other environment harming activities that amount to trillions of dollars in subsidies. Christiana Figueres, ex head of the UN climate change convention says, "Harmful subsidies must be redirected towards protecting the climate and nature, rather than financing our own extinction." If this is not upside-down, then I don't know what is.

Businesses Benefit, People Suffer

Eva Zabey, executive director of Business for Nature says, "Many businesses are benefiting from these environmentally harmful subsidies. This cannot be a taboo topic. We need to speak using facts and understand where the financial flows are going. . . . Typically, the subsidies were established with good intentions in mind. We need to level the playing field because right now, some are benefiting from a head start when it should be the other way round. It's a wicked problem." A UN report from 2021 found that almost 90% of farm subsidies are harmful to the environment and human health, and they are driving inequality by excluding the smaller farms. Head explosion emoji!!

How Can This Change?

Where is the will to change these policies? How will the majority ever overcome the minority? If the politicians are overtly corrupt. And the majority of citizens are too distracted, fogged up, busy, and slowed down. Plus overweight, addicted, and paranoid. Who benefits most?

Paranoia, sickness, fear and conspiracy are good business. Stay home and watch your TV. Buy, consume, take this pill to make the pain and fear go away. I will keep saying it: fear taps into the monkey brain. It stops rational thought. Fear is selling us into our collective demise. Getting clear headed will enable humanity to turn things right-side up. Clarified thinking will, at the very least, allow humans to think right-side up.

You May Have A Moral Fiber But Corporations And Politicians Don't

Zoom out and put yourself in "their" shoes. Start to think like corporations and politicians. Throw out any guardrails and preconceived ideas, ethics, and morals you may have. You personally may have an ethic or moral fiber, and that's a good thing.

Never assume that a mega corporation, whose only responsibility is profits for its shareholders. Or politicians, who are beholden to their donors, have any morals. None of them will, though they will pretend they do and repeatedly tell you so. Never, ever give a politician or corporation the benefit of the doubt.

The Tools Of The Trade

People in positions of power wield traditions, precedent, status quo, culture, religion, money, food, and fear as talking points. These things are actually the balls and chains of society attached by our rulers, holding humanity back. The worst part is that humans have convinced themselves they need to keep carrying on the same way to our own detriment.

Citizens vote against their futures and fund exactly what is not in their best interests. It is truly maddening. Get clear headed and see for yourself. With a clear, objective mind and some critical thinking skills, you will never be able to see the world the same way.

Though, I have to admit, it may be maddening to see the real world. Ignorance truly may be bliss here. At least until you get cancer or some other terminal illness. Or a hurricane, flood, heat wave or fire take your home and loved ones.

Manipulation 24/7 - 365 Days A Year

Every move in this life is scripted and tested. Humans are being manipulated 99% of the time we're awake. This life is manipulated 24/7, 365 days a year on repeat until we die. They know you much better than you know yourself.

The first step in fighting back is to get educated. Don't handicap yourself by giving power to the few. Accountability matters. No people in power should ever be given the benefit of the doubt. Not ever. Make them prove their words with actions.

Words Are Meaningless

Air is free, for now at least. Political speech cost them nothing. They work for us. That is their mandate. Make the politicians show citizens their sincerity with actions. Not fake word salad doublespeak, and definitely not with bills and laws that are named something good, yet actually achieve the polar opposite.

Do not even bother to listen to their lip service. They are speaking with the intention to manipulate you. Follow their actions and the money. Hold them accountable, for without accountability politicians will certainly flout any ambiguity, gray areas, loopholes, or benefit of doubt you provide them. This is already commonplace. We see daily how the laws that apply to the many are flouted by the few.

We The People have to be laying the groundwork for a new way to think about human society, life, health, yourself, and the world around you. It's so easy to be angry. Yet, humanity must learn to inspire love, kindness, understanding, and compassion. Not just competitive climbing on top of each other for money. It's a trick. Kindness, compassion and love are not weak traits, as those in power will have you believe. These are actually the traits of the strong.

Can You Ever Trust Someone Who Only Puts Money First?

Would you personally trust a person who puts money before everything else? Do you think you could rely on this person if an accident occurred? This hypothetical person will be calculating the cost of response to the accident and how they could spin the situation to benefit themselves.

What if you are hurt and you call on this person for help? They may have to spend time and money. In their head they are calculating the added cost of the opportunity to help you. Should they determine there is no personal benefit to helping you, then you may be stuck.

Altruism is not a part of the standard corporate or government charter. To the corporation, government, and politicians, added cost without benefit incentive is bad business. Yet, there is real value in caring and kindness. It's called self-worth.

What if making money first before anything else is written into this hypothetical person's operating code and procedure? This procedure places profits before everything and is signed and notarized. This is the truest definition of a corporation.

Corporations Are Not Your Friend

Mega corporations are not your friend. Although they will advertise friendliness to you. They'll tell you about all the great things they, as your friend, do on your behalf. Doing everything they can to make you feel warm and fuzzy. In reality, this is just to obfuscate.

Meanwhile, behind your back. They have a team lobbying against the very things they gleefully advertise to you that they're doing to help you.

To help the Earth, to help humanity. These human run corporations are opposite people too.

Would you personally trust a human who behaves and thinks in this manner? If a corporation holds the same legal standing as a human. Then why not treat this human run corporation with the same amount of skepticism you would show toward a snake oil salesman?

They All Know What They Are Doing

All politicians and corporations absolutely know the negative effects of their products and rhetoric. They only act ignorant because it's convenient. Because they know they have the benefit of the doubt given by kind, hard working, everyday people.

Why do citizens accept this two tier system? It is probably because people feel powerless. Or maybe think they are not smart enough and trust the gatekeepers more than those banging at the gates.

There really is a two tiered system. Guilty first until proven innocent for most. Innocent until proven guilty for the few. If you can pay for the lawyers, public relations firms, the media, and get your friends to write positive op-ed stories and change laws, anything can be spun to seem like a reasonable doubt.

Every day, citizens let the corporations and politicians get away with this doublespeak. It has come to a point where politicians will say just about anything, no matter how outlandish and untrue. As long as you donate to them and give them your vote, it will stay this way. Humanity has come to a point where we can no longer tolerate this business as usual.

The Powerful Are Not Better Than Anyone

It begs the question. Why do we give the fortunate the benefit of the doubt? Are they not just as flawed as every other human? Yet, with the means, connections, and power to carry out any of their wildest and darkest wishes.

Do we assume they must have some extra special sense of control over themselves, an altruism gene? Or, like they say, maybe we should assume their DNA is special. This is a collective mental problem. We have been conditioned throughout history to believe these larger than life humans are somehow superhuman and virtuous.

It's the others that are always trying to accuse them, smear them. They're just jealous and it's all fake news, they say. They just want my money and to bring me down. I didn't do it because I am so great. Trust me, don't trust my accusers. Blame the victims.

Now, I'm not saying the accusations and lawsuits are always frivolous. But sometimes it's just so obviously true and yet even still. Deny, deny, deny. I give to charity, and am a family man with kids.

I am a "maker," they say. They say "I create jobs." Pitting the so-called "takers" against each other like pawns. So easily distracted, people forget every little transgression and move on to the next red light flashing crisis in their own daily lives. I find it extremely difficult to believe this is all happening coincidentally.

More Upside-Down Trickery

Here is an interesting argument. Who is truly the maker and who is actually the taker? The verbiage is once again upside-down. Are the makers not the everyday people that work in the factories, shops, et cetera? The ones assembling cars, baking cakes, keeping the power on. Wouldn't it seem more correct to call working class citizens the makers? Without them, nothing would be, well, made.

Since the billionaire class, the politicians, and the corporations hire the best accountants and do as much as possible to avoid paying taxes, they certainly do not make things. They take from others to make things. For example taking the bank's money to work for them. Often they also receive grants and subsidies from the government. It's easy to get loans when you're rich. Where does the bank's money come from?

Apple did not invent the iPhone. A French software engineer named Jean-Marie Hullot did. Apple just paid to have it mass produced. So they could sell it and make profits. Do we need an iPhone? Humans existed millions of years without one.

If you start to think about what a smart phone in your pocket does. You might realize that even though you believe it is giving some sort of freedom. It's actually a tool of restriction and surveillance. We just haven't quite reached that point in the United States, yet. They have already arrived in China however.

A smartphone is a tool of connivence. What does it do? Naturally, it increases productivity. It also keeps us on a line. Not online, on a line. It's a camera, microphone and GPS device in our pocket. It records our conversation in texts. With it we are able to "share" our life with the rest of the world. Think about all the products and profits made from the invention of the smartphone. Fifteen years later we can't live without them. We are now dependent on them.

They Know You Better Than You Know Yourself

Politicians and corporations know you better than you know yourself. Every angle is covered. They have data points on all the citizens and group them into categories. They know just by the brands you buy what type of person you are. This is a fact.

These people manipulate the citizen muppets. Zombified in the matrices of a food chain and work culture built to make us sick and keep us unhealthy. Designed to keep us from thinking clearly. To keep people weak, afraid and taking their medications. To keep people consuming for the short lived gratification it brings. And the long term profits for those at the top.

They want us hanging on every word of political creation. Paranoid citizenry is good business. They sell conspiracy after conspiracy. Lie after lie. Nothing to see here. Continue to consume and debit. Be afraid and never have the time, or chance, to turn yourself right-side up.

Alcoholism Feeds Conspiracy

I'd like to add a bit of personal detail here and think it's pertinent in this context. I used to drink a lot of hard alcohol and beer. Then I stopped drinking alcohol for many years. And the effects are undeniable. During my heavy drinking years I was always paranoid and believing in all the latest conspiracies.

The funny thing that happened when I stopped drinking alcohol regularly. Was that all the conspiracy and paranoid delusions just stopped. It wasn't like the next day of course, it took a year to detox. But in the end the voices in my head just completely stopped.

Alcohol can, and does cause hallucinations. Not to mention the many other negative side effects on the human brain from alcohol. Who can say for sure the additional effects of chemical additives in beers, wine and liquors have on the mind. Besides truly inhibiting proper thinking and ruining your sleep.

After I stopped drinking alcohol. It made me think about how Americans tend to be very heavy drinkers. When I considered how many beers and hard liquors contain chemicals and corn syrup. I couldn't help but ponder that half the reason half of America is so paranoid is because they are not living in reality.

Everyday consumption of alcohol leads to a smaller brain size, depression, hallucinations, poor sleep and paranoia. When you get clean, you get clear. The paranoia and conspiracy disappear. All of a sudden what was once right-side up becomes clear that it's actually upside-down.

CHAPTER TWELVE

Keywords

English is an amazing language. Many languages are ambiguous. Based on ideas, metaphors, and inference of meaning. The specialty of English is being specific or not. One of the most beautiful traits about the English language is that it's ever changing. Creatively, this is a wonderful thing.

Language Is Amazing

As a kid in school, you must speak the slang and know the key words the kids are using. Each generation of innovation, creativity, and growth gives us new words and things to define. If you consider the undertaking to catalog, define, keep track of, and find the origin. To create a dictionary of every single word, it's quite a significant task.

Language is what has enabled humanity to build society to the point we are at today. We could not have come this far without speech and language. Who gave us language? Where did all these words come from? More on this in chapter 14.

I believe it is important to understand the concept of keywords, in more than one sense. One example of a very sinister use of keywords happening every day involves searching on the internet. In this example, I am specifically talking about what researchers call "endemic greenwashing."

Keyword Searches On The Internet

The Guardian analyzed ads served in search results on the most popular search engine. Working in collaboration with InfluenceMap, which is "a think tank that tracks the lobbying efforts of polluting industries." They conducted searches using 78 different climate related terms.

What they found was that more than 1 in 5 ads were "placed by companies with significant interests in fossil fuels." Banks, oil companies, and PR firms. These companies are buying ads that link to articles, which appear in search results, looking like regular information. So, when people are searching for climate change related information, these companies can frame and spoon feed the narrative in a way that benefits them. To influence how people think about the topic.

Simply speaking, the most popular search engine (and undoubtedly other search engines) are "letting groups with a vested interest in the continued use of fossil fuels pay to influence the resources people receive when they are trying to educate themselves."

Instead of "contesting the science," like the oil and gas companies did for decades, they now spin it. Contesting the science came to an end when the information came out in 2015 that oil companies have known the effects of their products on climate change since the late 1970s. Even though they knew, they continued to deny and promote misinformation for decades until it all came to public view in 2015.

People Can't Tell The Ads From Actual Search Results

Something to note. Another study in 2020 found that more than 50% of users reportedly could not tell the difference between these ads and the real search results. These companies are doing everything they can to make business as usual look like something else by influencing "discussions about decarbonization in their favor." How does this help the environment? How does this help us move away from being petroleum people? Naturally, it doesn't, and that's the point of course.

Nothing has changed. Today, they're instead trying to influence the information people find when they search it out themselves, obfuscating the true story. This practice is informational warfare at best and frankly gaslighting at worst. It's not only the information they put on the internet, but also the information they use in their annual reports. This approach leads to a total greenwashing of their activities.

Say One Thing Do The Opposite

"Until there is very concrete progress, we have every reason to be very skeptical about claims to be moving in a green direction," said Professor Gregory Trencher at Kyoto University in Japan. Trencher worked with Mei Li and Jusen Asuka at Tohoku University. In February, 2022, these researchers published a peer reviewed paper in PLOS ONE.

What they found is that major oil companies are all talk and no action when it comes to claims of transforming their businesses into more green models. Researchers found, "Financial analysis reveals a continuing business model dependence on fossil fuels along with insignificant and opaque spending on clean energy."

Further, the researchers state, "If they were moving away from fossil fuels we would expect to see, for example, declines in exploration activity, fossil fuel production, and sales and profit from fossil fuels," Professor Trencher said. "But if anything, we find evidence of the reverse happening."

This is just more opposite people talk, and is the gold standard: say one thing, do the opposite. "The companies are pledging a transition to clean energy and setting targets more than they are making concrete actions."

Money Always Does What Is In Money's Best Interests

The banks, PR companies, and oil companies have huge sums of money involved in the fossil fuels industries. This endless need and corruption seems impossible to stop. Unless humans get smart and become more forceful in our demands for change.

This is only one example. There are countless other industries doing exactly the same thing on the internet and with advertising. Not only that, they are printing it into books.

Children's Books

Starting in 2019 the American Farm Bureau has been publishing children's books under a publishing company called Feeding Minds Press. The American Farm Bureau is an arm of the agrochemical industrial farming lobby group called the American Farm Bureau Federation. More examples of a good sounding name with nefarious purposes.

According to an article in Vice, Big Agriculture Is Printing Children's Books That Say Pesticides Are Great. "The sprawling industrial farming operations represented by the Farm Bureau are one of the biggest polluters of freshwater in the U.S., and a major source of methane and nitrous oxide, two highly potent greenhouse gases. As recently as three years ago, the Farm Bureau was officially questioning if humans are causing the climate to warm (it's now partnering with corporate-friendly environmental groups and calling for "voluntary" industry-led climate solutions). The Farm Bureau is currently fighting with "energy and passion" an attempt by the Biden administration to bring in tougher regulations keeping pollution out of streams, rivers, lakes, and oceans."

"It's obviously nefarious," Jennifer Jacquet, an associate professor of environmental studies at New York University, told VICE News. "If you want to spread propaganda, starting with what we tell our children is a very good place to begin."

We are here now as a society. Do you think you can trust big business to do the right thing? This is the truest behavior of corporations and their lobbyists. Manipulation at its most precise. Convincing children, the very people who will suffer the most from the climate destruction. To keep on killing the environment. It's time to open our eyes to the truth.

Communication Enables Us To Fulfill Tasks

Let's look at the idea of keywords from a different perspective. Communication is what enables us to thrive. How could humans fulfill tasks if they were unable to speak to our counterparts? Or communicate needs? Look at your pet for example. Humans take visual cues from facial expressions and body language. Yet, one can't decipher any complex thoughts.

What is humanity's real purpose? Is there one? Is it producing and consuming? Why does it seem that the purpose of life is to fulfill tasks? Most Americans spend approximately more than 70% of their days each week, fulfilling tasks for others, to earn money, just to exist. To have shelter, food, and clothes. Many who have died and come back to life stated that they had further "work" to do. Likely meaning they had more tasks to fulfill. It wasn't the time for them to clock out, yet.

Is The Circuit Board Art Imitating Life, Or Life Imitating Art?

Is a circuit board the reflection of human civilization? Or are we the reflection of a circuit board? Doesn't a circuit board look exactly like a city with houses and roads? What happens in these 'houses' and 'roads' on a circuit board?

Tasks are fulfilled and data is moved from one place to another by electrons, little positive bits of energy. Look at an office building. What happens in an office building? Tasks, presumably, carried out by humans who are only .00001% matter—and 99.99999% bits of energy. In every building, home or office, humans complete tasks everyday. Then get in their car and travel from one task center to another.

Keywords As Trigger Functions

The deeper we dig into our subconscious. The more we learn that words and sentences suddenly become easily likened to strings of computer code, or commands. Executing and triggering behaviors, actions, emotions, responses, feelings, et cetera.

Only by becoming aware and able to acknowledge the existence of these pre-programmed reactions to keywords will we be able to help reprogram ourselves. We can do this by editing the strings of code that are triggered by advertisers, corporations and politicians. We must step out from the matrix in order to see inside it clearly.

Your Brain Is A Super Computer

Human brains could be said to be supercomputers. Running programs, conditioned to recognize keywords and catchphrases. If you are a brand or politician, then you learn to say the right keywords. The ones that tested well with the research panel. Like when you type into the search bar what's trending pops up first, your brain acts in a similar way.

When using specific keywords. What are the feelings, associations, and ideas the majority of the test subjects take away when using a certain phrasing? Do these strings of commands fulfill the messaging? Most importantly, will they stimulate a purchase or vote? Will they make humans do what we want them to do, feel, and think?

Framing Is Important

The next step taken in programming is framing. The use of the term "frame" means to frame an idea. Framing informs the context. In coding, brackets could be referred to as the frame. Inside these brackets are strings of code that execute the commands of the coder.

Choosing words carefully every day, humans paint a picture of our meanings. We frame them in a way that is appealing to others, or flattering to ourselves. Choosing words carefully we are executing subconscious programs in the minds of others to manipulate their behaviors. Advertisers, politicians and the media do this with scientific precision.

Framing Shapes Opinions

The most simple example is the left versus right programming in the media. The angle, headline, wordage, and framing of the "story." Will make a similar set of facts or even a quote, seem to mean something much different in the context given, or not given. So will the style of the presentation, whether it's written on a page or given live.

When in person humans read facial cues. When watching TV the human brain treats TV no different than when in person. The codes exist, and the unconscious programs are triggered, whether or not humans are consciously aware or in agreement.

Framing is stronger in informing us and shaping our opinions than we may be willing to accept. Our gut is telling us not to trust. Probably a lot. Yet, how can we trust our guts if the messages and signals have been hacked?

The First Story Is The One Most Likely To Be Believed

From a statistical and psychological standpoint, the first story a person hears is the one they tend to believe. That's why news is always "breaking." Whoever gets the story first. Gets to break the framing and context. Setting up how the story is shaped into memory as an original neurological signal and idea—the thought of the idea as presented in the context, left or right, good or bad.

Since humans, more often than not, search out information that feeds into biases, we tend to turn away from information that challenges beliefs. Instead, looking to affirming sources. This habit is just enforcing a feedback loop. In order to be objective, humans need to search out sources of information running contrary to their ideas and think critically.

Only looking to sources of affirming information is ensuring change of thought and objectivity will never happen. Further, by stating that any information from any other source is "fake" keeps the narrative in check. It's basic propaganda 101.

Objectively Viewing All Points Of View

I will read the right side view and the left side view. Usually, then I am able to make an informed, critically thought out decision. Yet, again this is only a decision made from information that is being fed to me. So what is the actual truth?

I experienced this first hand photographing the Occupy Wall Street protests. I was on the Brooklyn Bridge, at Wall Street, in Zuccotti Park. I even found myself, on the Brooklyn Bridge, in a wide angle photo on the cover of a magazine printed in England.

I had been uploading my photos online and was being contacted by organizations who wanted to publish them. Because I was taking pictures of all the "normal" people and was also in the thick of the action.

I found the New York Times only focused on, and ran photos of the weirdos, vagrants and the homeless people. Not only that, what they wrote was so different from what I experienced being there every day. They only presented it in a negative light.

The Echo Chamber... Chamber... Chamber

What if that's the plan all along? To keep people living in a feedback loop. Using informational warfare and groupthink to re-enforce the same idea. Manipulating people to make decisions that go against their own best interests.

It's not a what if, it's gaslighting, and it's happening every day in the Anthropocene. This type of informational warfare is not new. But it has gotten much worse and more prevalent in the internet and social media age.

Rejection Of Non-Confirming Information

For example, look at what happened to Fox News after the 2020 election. Suddenly, Fox News wasn't telling their viewers the information that they wanted to hear. So there was this big shift to alternative news sources. And Fox lost money!

Regular Fox viewers started claiming Fox wasn't good anymore. This is exactly my point above. In this situation there is almost no chance of changing this type of person's views, regardless of new information or facts. They only want to hear affirming viewpoints. Which makes me wonder how many people will actually read this book cover to cover?

In a court of law, the judge and jury have two opposing sides. They argue with as much fact, expert opinion and data available to prove their respective points. This could be referred to as equitable justice.

Judges are trained to think and see critically. There are specific rules they must follow. They weigh the merits of each side and attempt to separate spin, obfuscation, framing, and bias in search of "truth," using evidence. Humans need to become impartial judges and learn all of the tricks being used against them and search for the evidence.

Critical thinking and objectivity are two of the most important skills every human can learn. Another skill to learn is to be able to separate your personal emotion and bias from the information at hand.

CHAPTER THIRTEEN

Detox

Everyday we make judgments, unconsciously and consciously. Sometimes we make ill informed decisions built on top of judgements and biases, based upon feelings and emotions. Yet, how could we truly be in touch with our feelings when pretty much everyone is never actually clear headed?

One may think they are clear headed. Or level headed. Yet, how could this be if the pure message is clouded by toxins? In our food, air, water, and more. Do you drink coffee? Alcohol? Eat at restaurants? Sleep in a bed? Sit on a couch? Use cosmetics, shampoo? Smoke cannabis? Always get a good night's sleep? Have money stress? Kids? Not to mention the chemicals sprayed on and contained in most everyday foods. The list goes on, and on, and on.

Everyday Toxins Are Affecting Your Emotions, Thoughts And Decisions

The human brain is very emotionally fallible. Do you personally control every single one of your inputs? Do you know how many chemicals are in that beer, the air you breathe, or in your food? What about the pharmaceuticals, added coloring and preservatives in your fish? Are you aware that MSG (monosodium glutamate) is not just for Chinese restaurants? Many regular restaurants, as well as Michelin Starred restaurants, consider MSG an important ingredient in their dishes.

How about which of the thousands of additives, phthalates, and chemicals have been approved to be in your food, detergent, furniture, cosmetics, shampoo, clothing, toys, et cetera. Do you know which chemicals are in your tap water? How about the chemicals that leach from the pipes they flow in?

Do you think meat can make people depressed and/or aggressive? Imagine the negative energy associated with a slaughterhouse. How about the antibiotics, hormones, and ractopamine inside that meat. What about how those chemicals affect your thoughts day to day? Can you say for certain you know how all of these chemicals, additives, and preservatives affect human brain and body functions? You can't. It's simply impossible for you to know. Unless you cut them all out.

The Facts Regarding Meat Are Stark

Meat is very political and the facts are stark. If you are unaware, ractopamine is a chemical used to increase lean muscle growth in animals. Ractopamine is banned from use in 160 countries. According to the NIH "ractopamine is fed to an estimated 80% of all beef, swine, and turkey raised in the United States. It promotes muscle mass development, limits fat deposition, and reduces feed consumption." In other words ractopamine increases profits!

"However, it has several undesirable behavioral side effects in livestock, especially pigs, including restlessness, agitation, excessive oral-facial movements, and aggressive behavior." Pigs happen to be very smart and share genetic traits with humans. This is what makes it possible for pig-to-human heart transplants. So if ractopamine is having these effects on pigs. I'd say there's a better chance than not that consuming ractopamine is going to have similar negative effects on humans.

Just Like Humans Animals Are Energy

Since most people are far removed from their food. They are not aware of the traumas animals endure due to how they are raised and killed. Just like humans, animals are .00001% matter and 99.9999% energy.

Growing up I hunted deer with my father. Many times you have to track the animal and often put it out of its misery with your knife. Every time I shot a deer and it was still breathing when I found it. I could see the fear in their eyes. It's something you don't forget.

Do you think a massive animal like a cow or a pig is not aware of what's going on? Sure, it's convenient to be ignorant. To think that these animals are dumb and don't have emotions or intelligence. Only you would be mistaken to make such a false assumption. All animals have natural instinct, personalities, feel fear and have feelings. Any pet owner will attest to this.

Do you think the animals that you eat are happy when they die? Did this animal live a happy healthy life? Not likely, if 80% of beef and 70% of pork is coming from four corporations. From a purely energetic standpoint, when you eat meat, you are consuming the sorrow, stress, sadness, and associated hormones of that animal. Not to mention all of those added chemicals and antibiotics. This statement is backed by science.

Meat Is A Big Destructive Business

For more perspective on meat eating. Beef is a $30 billion industry per year in America. In countries like Australia, America, and Spain, on average, citizens are consuming in excess of 100 kilograms / 220 pounds of meat each year.

Livestock grazing and feed production occupies 27% of Earth's landmass. For comparison, human settlements occupy only 1% and forests account for 26%. Humans are dedicating more than one quarter of the Earth's surface solely for the purpose of raising animals to kill and eat them.

Not only that, it takes 15,500 liters / 4095 gallons of water to produce each kilogram / 2.2 pounds of beef. Each year, more greenhouse gasses are produced from beef farming than the entire worldwide transportation sector.

Think about the massive amount of negative energy and waste that goes into this system. The scale is so large it is pretty much unimaginable to comprehend. This industry is incredibly polluting to the Earth, body, and mind.

Eating Meat Is Addictive

I personally used to love eating grilled porterhouse and ribeye steak. But after I stopped eating meat, I stopped craving it. Once in a while I find myself in a situation where my choices are extremely limited and I end up eating some meat.

Usually, if I eat more than a few bites, the next day I wake up feeling depressed and less energetic. Meat is not only addictive, it is also a depressant in my case. However, when I was eating meat regularly it made me aggressive. It made me aggressive to the point where I noticed it.

There's studies that show optimal performance for athletes actually comes from eating meat free diets. Even Arnold Schwarzenegger and NFL athletes agree on these benefits. On the down-side, studies have shown that meat eating can decrease penis size and increase erectile dysfunction. Yup, those are the down-side effects.

All the hormones, chemicals, and antibiotics getting pumped into these animals. To make them grow fast and stay healthy in cramped living quarters. Are mixing a meat cocktail ripe to alter clearheadedness and behavior. Not to mention the long term detrimental effects to your health, the environment, and society.

Food Is Very Political

It's no wonder that meat is a part of the culture wars. There are so many entrenched monetary interests in this sector. How could it not be political? Humans have to recognize that food is much more political, energetic, and contaminated than can be imagined. Meat farming is also destroying the environment.

Looking at food is the first step toward getting a clear view of the area you inhabit. The saying goes, "You are what you eat." If everything humans eat, drink and breath are toxic. How could we not be toxic humans?

The last decade has brought into focus how important gut health is to everything. It's now more out in the open than ever how our current system of refined foods, added sugars, antibiotics, and chemical additives destroy gut health and the overall health of our bodies and minds.

Most people will argue. The FDA, USDA and EPA say it's OK! To that statement I pose this question. Do the chemical companies, meat producers, and agricultural corporations give money to the people who make the laws that govern them? We all know the answer is unequivocally yes.

Does the American government do a cost benefit analysis before implementing regulations? As I explained in chapter 11, we know they do. Right in front of our eyes everyday, the politicians, government officials, and corporations show us how corrupt, lacking in will, and inept they are.

About 90,000 Different Chemical Are Dumped Into Sewers Each Year

I would need to write a twenty volume encyclopedia in order to detail all of the chemicals and the effects of these chemicals on human health and psychology. According to the Sierra Club, somewhere in the neighborhood of 90,000 different man-made chemicals are discharged into our sewers each year. In order to see why we need to completely eliminate chemicals from the loop, we have to understand how they keep harming us residually.

One of the largest sources of residual chemical pollution comes in the form of biosolids, which is just a fancy way of saying sewage sludge. In the United States, sewage sludge is not only composed of human waste but also waste from factories, slaughterhouses, industrial facilities, and other businesses that legally discharge waste directly into the sewage system.

Taxpayers subsidize this because tax dollars pay for the treatment of sewage. In the European Union there is legislation that places the onus on industry to deal with and manage their chemical waste. It is time for America to enact similar legislation. Since politics and money control everything in America. We The People will have to seriously pressure the politicians to hold industry accountable.

Biosolids

The EPA (Environmental Protection Agency) states that approximately 50% of American sewage waste is "treated" and then used to fertilize croplands. Remember, as I mentioned in chapter 9, pharmaceuticals are not considered contaminants and therefore are not removed from sewage. Neither are PFAS.

According to Science Direct, the United States produces around 12.7 million tons of dry municipal sewage waste (biosolids) per year. That means biosolids use is somewhere in the neighborhood of five or six million tons per year. For reference, the entire world produces approximately 1.3 billion tons per year.

Biosolids Are Used To Fertilize Crops

What happens when dry sewage waste is used to grow crops? Pharmaceuticals and "forever chemicals" like a 9,000+ subset of chemicals called PFAS (Perfluoroalkyl and Polyfluoroalkyl substances) are being put into the soil, the crops growing from that soil, the animals that eat those crops, and the groundwater. This class of chemicals is called forever chemicals because they don't degrade or break down. Not ever.

According to the NIH, PFAS "keep food from sticking to cookware, make clothes and carpets resistant to stains, and create firefighting foam that is more effective. PFAS are used in industries such as aerospace, automotive, construction, electronics, and military." In June 2022 the EPA released a report stating that there are no safe levels for human consumption of PFAS. Current peer-reviewed scientific studies have shown that exposure to PFAS may lead to:

• Reproductive effects such as decreased fertility or increased high blood pressure in pregnant women

• Developmental effects or delays in children, including low birth weight, accelerated puberty, bone variations, or behavioral changes

• Increased risk of some cancers, including prostate, kidney, and testicular cancers

• Reduced ability of the body's immune system to fight infections, including reduced vaccine response

• Interference with the body's natural hormones

• Increased cholesterol levels and/or risk of obesity

These are just the peer reviewed studies listed on the government edited website. We already know how the government controls the flow of information. Who really knows how many side effects and health hazards there are from this class of chemicals. And this is just one single class of chemicals in biosolid waste.

Why Doesn't The EPA Do Something?

In a 2018 report, the EPA office of inspector general said the EPA couldn't regulate biosolids because "it lacked the data or risk assessment tools needed to make a determination on the safety of 352 pollutants" found in biosolid samples. They lack the data and tools to make a determination on just 352 chemicals of 90,000! This is government reasoning: "we can't figure it out (throws hands up in the air), all well." And so business as usual continues, contaminating the environment and human health so corporations can keep making money.

It's Not Biosolid Use That Is The Problem

The use of biosolids in agriculture has been going on for hundreds of years or more. Using biosolids as a natural fertilizer is a great way to amend the soil and to use regenerative practices. It is not the usage that is bad. Just like with everything, ingredients matter, inputs matter.

Reusing human waste is the most effective and efficient way to dispose of it. However, in order to keep doing it, there needs to be a proper system and regulation in place. Those 90,000 different types of chemicals that are being dumped into American sewers each year, have to be kept from getting into the sewage waste in the first place. Companies need to be held accountable and take responsibility. There is no way around food being political. Next to water, food is our most important input.

The Chemicals In Our Environment

PFAS are all around us every day. They are in our cosmetics, furniture, shampoo, toothpaste, cooking utensils, rain gear, food wrappers, and even our dental floss. One study indicated PFAS chemicals are in 98% of all Americans' blood.

In 2019, researchers tested breast milk and found that every one of the women tested had PFAS in their breast milk. I repeat, PFAS are endocrine and hormone disruptors. Babies born in the 21st century are already contaminated from birth. Directly from their mother's milk.

This doesn't account for the micro plastics found in plastic baby bottles, sperm and food packaging.

Contaminated Beef

In February, 2022, the Michigan Department of Agriculture and Rural Development issued an advisory. Beef from a local farm had high levels of PFOS, which is part of the group of chemicals referred to as PFAS.

The farm had been growing crops to feed their cattle, using biosolids as fertilizer for these crops. This is only one small, yet very clear example where biosolid waste has contaminated crops. Imagine, there are six million tons of biosolid waste being used each year to fertilize crops.

Crops that not only humans eat, but also birds, bugs, ducks, deer, pigs, turkeys, pheasants, quail, cows, sheep, goats, chickens, gophers. Every animal that lives within that ecosystem. Additionally, the wastewater from these farms runs off into groundwater, streams and rivers. So even if you think you are catching a wild "clean" duck, deer, turkey or fish, chances are you are not.

Some More Examples

Now we see how contaminated our waste and agricultural system is, let me share a few more examples of how these chemicals get into our bodies and eliminated into the environment. Here are some lesser known FDA "OK" additives in food that are banned in other countries.

Farm raised salmon is fed astaxanthin (a petrochemical) to make its flesh the coral color. This coloring in wild salmon comes naturally from eating krill. It would be hard to sell farm raised salmon, as salmon, if it had white flesh. Instead they fake it.

Another is BVO, brominated vegetable oil. It's used as an emulsifier in sodas. BVO prevents the separation of ingredients. It also happens to be used in flame retardants. BVO can build up in the human body and cause skin and nerve damage as well as memory loss. These chemicals are also eliminated from your body into the sewage system.

Others are endocrine and hormone disruptors like BHT, Butylated hydroxytoluene, a cousin of BHA, butylated hydroxyanisole. BHA has been shown to lower testosterone and sperm counts in rats. Both are flavor enhancers and preservatives suspected to cause cancer.

One will find BHA and BHT in everything from cereal, butter, chewing gum, stuffing mix and sausage links, to crackers, pie crusts and cosmetic creams. Another preservative shown to be an endocrine disruptor is propylparaben, used in creams, cosmetics, shampoos, and bath products, to name a few. Which, we wash down the drain when showering and bathing.

Then there are phthalates. Phthalates are in toys, vinyl flooring and wall coverings, detergents, lubricating oils, food packaging, pharmaceuticals, blood bags, and tubing. In addition to personal care products like nail polish, hair sprays, aftershave lotions, soaps, shampoos, perfumes, and other fragrances. Phthalates are also endocrine and hormone disruptors.

I couldn't make this select list without including nitrates and nitrites. These are used in cured meats and hotdogs and have been linked to stomach cancer. My father loved his sandwich meats and hot dogs.

My Experience With BHA

In an interesting turn of events. I am able to provide firsthand analysis, from my own personal experience with BHA and propylparaben. I had a fungal infection and tried as many holistic therapies as I could. Yet, I was still not able to completely clear this fungal infection. Left with no choice, I went to see a doctor.

I never go to the doctor and haven't even taken an aspirin in probably 15 years. I am fortunate to have a strong immune system and rarely get sick. The doctor prescribed an antifungal cream. I thought OK, this shouldn't be too bad. It is only a cream to put on my skin.

When I picked up the prescription there were quite a few odd side effects. One happened to be impotence. In one sense this surprised me. At the same time, the list of adverse effects did not surprise me. Since pharmaceuticals are known for their long lists of side effects.

However, the one side effect that jumped out at me the most, besides impotence, was depression. When I searched online I couldn't find any links that gave me the same list of side effects. Which I think is odd. I thought how can a cream for my skin cause depression? Then I forgot about it.

Since I stopped drinking alcohol, normally, I don't feel depressed. Living has its ups and downs. Usually, these periods do not last so long.

About two days into using this cream I started feeling really depressed, much more than I would usually, and for absolutely no reason. After a week I started to lose motivation to do things. Initially, I was stumped. Then, like a bolt of lightning, I realized it's the cream.

I used this cream for four weeks. For the entire period I was incredibly depressed to the point I was feeling like what's the point of doing anything. I couldn't get motivated. Two days after I stopped using this cream. Like a switch I was feeling much better. After a week I felt back to normal. I am still shocked at how much it changed my personality. I find this experience very unsettling. In the end I found the rash was not a fungal infection but was diet oriented!

Finding The Cause

The first thing I always do is read the ingredients of everything. I was reluctant to use this cream when I first got it. But I was feeling like my choices were limited. The first ingredient listed at 20% of the volume was the pharmacological agent that kills the fungus. The second ingredient, BHA. A few more fillers and then propylparaben, with water at the end.

If you are unfamiliar, when listing ingredients on packaging they are listed by weight. Simply put, the most is first and the least is last. This cream was 80% preservatives and fillers! The same exact preservatives they put in food and cosmetics. BHA and propylparaben—both endocrine and hormone disruptors.

If you are thinking maybe it was the antifungal agent. I don't believe it could be. Because I asked the doctor to prescribe a different antifungal cream without the preservatives. Not only did it not list depression as a side effect. I felt no adverse effects from using it.

Labeling For Food

When listing ingredients on a box of cereal, there is no law that requires the producer to list possible side effects. However, on a pharmaceutical they must. Here is some direct correlation that these preservatives can cause depression and potentially impotence.

Yet, here is proof of depression as listed by the side effects that I experienced firsthand. This cream also gave me rather large acne in areas near where I was using it. I have zero tolerance for these types of preservatives because I do not eat processed foods. So I am probably more sensitive than most.

The Chemical Makers Know The Adverse Effects

This brings full circle how the companies that supply these preservatives know exactly that they can cause depression and have many other negative side effects. They will still happily put them into food and other products that humans use internally and externally.

This helps to create another profit generating problem for them to solve. Making humans depressed is big business. Pharmaceutical companies are happy to sell antidepressants to fix depression. It's a very twisted way to be. Freedom is a chemical free existence.

Why Do We Trade Our Health For Convenience?

Why are humans giving their sanity, health, and trust simply to become addicts? To be surrounded with food and products that make us sick. Why are we giving up health and sanity for convenience, preservation, and artificial flavors?

These production methods favor the major corporations so they can mass produce and ship everywhere. Prolonging shelf life, generating massive profits, creating addiction. This is a reason why buying fresh and local is key to maintaining a healthy diet. And changing the current status quo.

We Voluntarily Give Our Health Away

Citizens are letting politicians, who have decided it was in their best interest, to govern us. And corporations, who's sole motive is the search for profits. To dictate what is food and what is not food.

Why do humans give these people and businesses the benefit of the doubt? Why do humans let ourselves believe doing this is OK? Because they use the "best words"? Or because the FDA says it is OK? Because it is convenient? Because the taste is so good? Because we are addicted and lazy?

Clear Thinking Requires Clean Inputs

Our big monkey brains are so easily manipulated. So easily short circuited. There is only one way to get clear headed: remove all inputs that are not the most basic of foods, clean air, and pure spring water. Get to know each and every one of your inputs—learn how and where they were produced. Know each ingredient. Learn how each one affects you when you consume it. It's that simple.

Real food is organically grown vegetables, greens, grains, nuts, and fruits. Spring water comes from a very deep and properly tested source. The freshest, cleanest air possible is to be found in areas with lots of trees. There are so many particulates in the air. Making it nearly impossible to find true clean air. It's also next to impossible to avoid microplastics. Scientists have found micro plastics in the most remote places on Earth and your bodies.

Detoxing Takes A Long Time And Is Not Fun

I will not soften the blow. It will take a long time to detox your body. There will be a significant amount of suffering from cravings, boredom, healing crises, and withdrawals. Having experienced this myself, I can tell you firsthand.

Combine this lifestyle with mindfulness and meditation because you have to control your thoughts as well as your future self's actions. You will absolutely come to the same realizations written in this book. It is like removing a veil and seeing the world around you clearly for the first time. These days when I walk around the supermarket, all I am able to see is twenty-four isles of sugar coated poisons.

Lifestyle Detox

This lifestyle detoxification is the closest we can ever come to "normal" or natural. Everything else is a manipulation. Like a scale, the environment, our food, and society is set up to drift us away from proper balance and calibration.

We keep living this way because it is all we have ever known. We need to reset, recalibrate, and learn to think again—this time without bias and without being manipulated. Detoxing is seeing things for what they are: a total and complete manipulation.

True Freedom

To be free, we must first control our thoughts. Second, we must have and maintain very strong willpower. Third, we must reconnect with empathy. With the collective energy of love, kindness, humanity, and the collective mind.

We have been convinced that stepping on top of and manipulating others is the way to live and get ahead. Who gave us these notions? The upside-down and opposite people. They want us to chase money and to be consumers at all costs. To keep having babies and make the GDP forever expand in the never ending search for more—more power, more control, more money. More to consume. More to buy and wield as a show of our status.

We must remove the ego from the decision making processes and commit to a life of less. Others will mock us at first. These are the ones who cannot control their own lives. They must attempt to control others. Deep down, chances are that they are afraid to confront themselves.

Once they see the greatness and change this way of living brings about in their peers, then they too will want the same for themselves. Don't belittle them for mocking you at first. Just lead by example. Show them kindness and greatness. They will think they are missing out. It's simple human psychology.

I've experienced this cycle first hand with my friends. First, they mocked me. Then they became inquisitive and eventually they followed my lead. All I did was stay strong, smile and lead by example. That's all it takes.

Cultivating Willpower

What is needed more than ever is individual willpower. Willpower to overcome money, peer pressure and the will of others trying to control you. To make you conform for their own personal gratification, not yours. Making themselves feel better about their lack of willpower.

You will find this power through meditation, diet, discipline, and exercise. You'll find willpower through putting your health and sanity first, before money. Through mental transcendence to be one with the web of life that is all around us.

Teach Kids To Meditate

We should be doing the same thing the pesticide companies are doing. Start with the kids. Changing thinking patterns from youth is the best first step to change the paradigm. The simplest and fastest way to change our society would be to implement daily meditation in all schools K-12. Dedicating one full hour daily to mindfulness practices and philosophy. This would seem such a simple idea with enormous benefits for society.

Yet, believe it or not, there have been K-12 schools that tried to implement meditation as a part of the curriculum, but Christian parents protested. Afraid that they may lose control over the minds of their young ones.

These parents called meditation and ideas of mindfulness "religion." When even Buddhists don't call Buddhism a religion. But rather a philosophy of living. Christian parents probably worry their children might come to their own conclusions and make decisions outside of the home.

These parents made such a stink that the schools stopped their efforts. The fear of mental freedom is strong in religion. The will to make the world a better place must be stronger. Many studies show that religion decreases rational and analytical thinking.

Don't Meditate, But Sugar And Pharmaceuticals Are OK

Often the same religious parents have no problems giving their children medication and letting them eat processed foods, sugar laden cereals, sodas, and corn syrup. Which, to me, doesn't make much sense. I say, take the "c" out of medication and replace it with a "t"—turning medication into meditation.

In many cases meditation can be a stronger form of healing than medication. This has been proven over and over again. There are many examples of people healing their bodies simply through mind control. I was even able to do this myself.

Get Kids Of Sugar

While on the subject of children, I'd like to state that the second simplest way to make change in society. Get kids off sugar. It should be illegal to have such an addictive substance in any kids' foods.

Yet, all kids' foods are filled with sugar. Get them off the easy, pre-packaged products, processed foods, sodas, snacks, and cereals. Most cereals contain BHT and or BHA and sodas have BVO. That should be reason enough, let alone the insane amounts of sugar in each product. Corporations want to hook kids as soon as possible so they can create lifelong addicts from as early an age as possible. They want to own your serotonin. They want to control your reward system. And once they do, you are an addict.

Why do you think all of the kids' products are full of sugar and sweeteners? If I were a parent, I would be trying to teach my kids good eating and life forming habits from the youngest age.

There is no parent that would let their kids get hooked on cocaine. Why the disconnect here? Why would parents let their kids get hooked on sugar? There is a reason kids always want sweets. It's because they are addicted. It is as simple as that. Children literally are the future. Let's teach them to be the change we want to see.

CHAPTER FOURTEEN

Honesty

What you give, you receive. With an objective mind, one may read this statement and find an example in their life where this is proven. Call it Karma. The law of reciprocity. An equal and opposite reaction. Boiled down, the idea is always the same.

If you are giving and kind, the saying goes, you will attract those kinds of people. If you are mean willed and spiteful, you will then indeed receive mean will and spitefulness from others. Treat others the same way they treat us. If we want trust, give trust and be trustworthy.

Retaliation Is Never The Answer

Think about gang violence, or the current political climate, it's all about reciprocity, retaliation, and revenge. Yesterday, the US black listed Chinese companies. Today, China blacklisted US companies. The more we poke each other in a negative direction. The more the needle will move into negative territory and the more we will all suffer.

One reason this is happening is because no one is willing to admit when they are wrong. Never owning a mistake. Humans want to act in any way they deem justifiable to themselves with impunity. To preserve an agenda, these people must maintain "face" and must keep up the appearance of strength.

What ever happened to taking the high road? It seems the high road has been closed for some time. With mindfulness and lifestyle changes, we will all be able to move beyond this upside-down world. Acts of kindness will inspire further acts of kindness. To be strong mentally is admitting when you are wrong. Not taking a defensive posture.

It's A Cliché - Yet It's True

Love is truly the answer. Psychologically speaking, humans that are lashing out have some mental issues. They are choosing this course of action from preformed subconscious neurological responses. Built upon a mechanism triggered by some past trauma or drama and a need for control and/or love.

Our society and its manipulative effects on the human brain are devastatingly clear. We tend to complain loudest about others, often projecting from that which we hate most in ourselves. Humans at the end of the day just want to be loved, accepted, and treated with kindness.

Who Wants Others To Be Mean To Them?

Seriously, who doesn't want people to be nice to them? Yet, kindness is often received with suspicion. This is a major side effect of upside-down world thinking. If a person says they want people to be mean to them, or says that all humans should be unkind to their fellow humans. Then there is some psychological and/or cultural damage there.

Society has built these massive metaphorical walls and rules that act like mental torture devices. In turn, humans have built defenses inside ourselves. There is this giant repressive structure built around money and nonsensical rules. Defining what we should be or how we should act.

Society Manipulates At The Behest Of Those In Power

The proverbial "They" have set our futures for us. Humanity just goes along because it's what everyone else does. Everyone wants to "get theirs." This is an incredibly short sighted way to think. Society is an extremely manipulative force and it doesn't benefit the majority of people when used in this manner.

From billionaire bullying and power moves, cultural machismo, to the most basic neighborhood gossip. The guardrails are calibrated by those in power for behavioral malfeasance. Humans trying to exert control over other humans. This is as old as civilization, and then some. Why do we care so much that we want to control other people so badly? Money, power, weakness, greed, ego, attention? Probably all of the above.

Stop Working For Free

Social media is a fine example. Its main proponent says that he just "wants to connect people." Yes, he wants to connect people to control them, their data, and the world. Of course this last bit is not being said out loud. But he's collecting your data, selling it, and enriching himself. One scandal after another follows him around like a plague. Every day, every time you log on, you are working for this person. For free.

Let me rephrase this. By using social media you are personally enriching the already wealthy by working for them for free! You are the product being sold. Work for free to be abused, taken advantage of, advertised to, lied to, and bullied by others on the platform. The cost of opportunity for the average person on social media is definitely not worth it.

Quit Social Media You Will Be Happier

We were more connected before social media. Social media has actually been shown to be tearing us further apart. Again, it's the upside-down world. Work for free. Get abused. Tear apart the fabric of society. All in the name of "connecting people." The cost outweighs the benefit here. Social media has metastasized into a cancer on society. The negative effects are obvious and the studies prove the harmful effects.

It's like a bad drug. Quit social media and see for yourself. After I left social media, it truly did improve my level of happiness and connectedness. Free yourself from working for free for those who are already wealthy.

Religion As An Institution Is Dishonest

Another example of a dishonest business is organized religion, which, by the way, is infallible. It sits high up on its pedestal. Beyond criticism. I'm not saying that all religious believers are bad people. Rather that religion is a tool for power and repression.

Religion as a whole has been used as a means to control, suppress and divide people since its inception. Every day preachers tell humans what to do and how to live. Policing others actions and thoughts with bullying, hate and ostracization. Religion always wants to convert you, for you to join them. To be like them. They even used to kill you if you didn't covert. Religion never stops trying to convince you. Always forcing their way, their view, on everyone else. They want you to live by their strict rules. Growing up Catholic, I can still feel the guilt.

Giving humans great justification to virtue signal, marginalize and to fight over whose religion is stronger or better. To subjugate or kill any who do not profess their loyalty. Always available, a religion that will tell you, what you want God, to want you to be. To confirm your misogyny, political views, or even your need to be rich and powerful.

Supplying unalienable powers to those who preach the gospel of God and the wonders of their divinity, with words from an unquestionable source. Just mention the code words, Jesus, God, Allah or any of the other deities to activate your power over others.

Religion Is An Excuse For Bad Behavior

When a "chosen" vessel takes part in criminal or unjust things. Just say "God uses imperfect people to do his perfect work." An easy justification and get out of jail free card for the self selected "chosen." Religion as an institution only cares about two things, money and power. Religion is not democratic.

Religion is an authoritarian excuse for those in power to call themselves the chosen ones. To say they are vessels of God. Therefore, no matter what imperfections are performed, the self chosen will simply say, they are performing the work of "God." Pitting their followers against everyone else to create division.

Religion is a wonderful, inscrutable, grift. That uses the power of fear to divide and subjugate. While raising up those in power, supporting top down hierarchies. All the while managing religion's justification to limit individualism and critical thinking.

Separating Businesses From Non-Profits

The first step to recognizing that religion, for the most part, is a grift, will be to take away the non-profit status of religious organizations that are not truly charities. Treating these so-called churches, real estate businesses and consultants like any other corporation or business. This will at least provide a small amount more accountability than they have now.

All connections between religion and politics need to be completely severed. The separation of church and state needs to be definitive, not gray like it is now. If you want to be religious, that is totally fine. But you don't get to push it on others, or use it to convince voters of your supposed "virtue." It's just tribalism in a suit.

These "chosen" prophets, as they like to call themselves, stand at podiums and in houses of worship telling people how to act, what to think, who to vote for, and what to believe or not believe. Merely selling people into being sheep. For themselves—self elected wolves—to prey on.

No need to think for yourself when religion thinks for you. Just like in chapter 10. When schools tried to implement meditation. Religious parents, who are totally fine telling others how to behave, think, and live. Find meditation is bad. It's just another great example of the hypocrisy of the controlling upside-down world. Graze with the flock. Be a follower and act like everyone else. Don't learn anything new. The words are infallible. The All Mighty Infallible.

The All Mighty Infallible

The All Mighty Infallible what? Humans have no idea. We have seen the never ending negative consequences of organized religion over, and over again, throughout history.

Humans hate because a book says so. Repress women and discriminate because a book says so. Kill and start wars in the name of religion. Seems more that it's an excuse to be intolerant and subjugate others. How can we even relate to the words in books written thousands of years ago? Written, chances are, with good intent but then co-opted by those in power to enforce hierarchical social structures, to control using fear.

Religion Is Groupthink At Its Worst

So much has changed in this time since these books were written. Humanity is so much more sophisticated and "educated." Still, the sheep will follow. It is easy. It is groupthink at its most efficient.

The manipulation must end and we must reset the paradigm. Religion has been shown to turn off rational thought in the brain of worshipers. Exactly what those in power want. Just do, don't think, or question our power.

A study by researchers from the University of British Columbia suggests that when analytical thinking rises religious beliefs drop. The time has come to discard what is holding us back from progress and from thinking and acting analytically.

What is interesting about this study. It also showed people who follow intuition more are more likely to believe in God. For me this is an odd juxtaposition.

Being Raised Roman Catholic

I obviously reject organized religion as an institution. Yet, I often follow my intuition. I do believe in energy. But not in one infallible, top down, almighty God telling us what to do. We are all energy. We are all God in the way that we are all one and connected.

I was raised Roman Catholic. Communion, catholic school, altar boy and all that jazz. Sit, stand, kneel, pray, feel guilty about everything. I'll never forget Sunday school. I despised it so much. Before class one day I hid in the woods. My father was looking and calling out for me. I waited until dark to come home. That was the last time my father ever tried to make me go to Sunday School.

What If It Was The Devil Who Wrote The Religious Texts?

In my opinion, if there is a Devil, a great and masterful demon, then he is surely a man. The man who wrote the books. Follow this train of thought with me. How many humans have killed other humans in the name of religion? Is not taking the life of another human being the supposed path to hell?

Hundreds of millions of souls, maybe even billions, have been killed, tortured, slaughtered, discriminated against, all in the name of religion. The first trick of the con man is to give confidence (faith) to the mark. The mark being the one to be conned. In my opinion this would make religion the most genius con ever. It's also a perfect part of the upside-down story.

The Negative Energy Associated With Religion Is Immense

Look at the numerous sex scandals of the church. For thousands of years this has been happening. The grooming and sexual molestation of young children. See how politicians wield religious affiliation as justification for misdeeds, wars and discrimination. How about the crusades, the Spanish inquisition, Jihad, extremism and fanaticism. The oppression and discrimination of women and honor killings. These are all products of religion.

There is an unending supply of examples where religion has been used as a means to suppress people. Still to this day. When you add it all up. It would seem the world would be a better place without religion. I'm not sure there is anyone who can argue that organized religion has done more good than bad for humanity. But I am sure some will try.

What Faith Really Is

Having faith, to me, is not reading and repeating a religious book. It's not believing in, or living religious words. Kneeling, singing hymns, saying Hail Marys, putting money in a basket, doing what a preacher tells us, attending mass on Sundays, or at whatever time of day, everyday bowing and praying to one single, top down ruler called God.

This top down philosophy is here to enforce current and past socio-economic norms. One big boss controls everyone else. This methodology works great for Emperors and Kings who were perceived to be gods by unknowing and uneducated peasants. Haven't we moved past this as a species by now?

Faith, in my opinion, is simply a faith born from goodness. Like I said earlier, what you give is what you receive. Religion does preach this, but the current and historical actions of the professed religious don't seem very pious to me.

Having faith is not believing in one God so you get into "Heaven" for an eternal life. This idea makes me think that those who want to live forever are simply afraid of death. It's not believing in, or kissing up to, one big boss. So you will get promoted to eternal life, or get eighty virgins in the afterlife—which by the way, seems really strange and perverted if you ask me. It's an odd reason to be religious, especially if you are a woman.

Faith is feeling comfort in the understanding that we are all energy and god. That you are a good person, because you are actually a good person. That we serve a greater purpose. Not to serve God, but to serve our energetic evolution. Not to be craven addicts chasing after everything we crave.

Waking up every day with a positive attitude, doing good deeds for others. Not just doing bad things and then going to God to ask for forgiveness. So you can do more bad things and not feel bad about it. Being a good person in the present is better than searching and bowing for an afterlife.

Things Do Happen For A Reason

Most things happen for a reason. In my opinion much of the reason why we are alive is to learn and grow from our past mistakes. Life is simple: try, fail or succeed, analyze, learn and repeat.

Throughout my life I have made many mistakes. And almost always, like a pendulum, people or circumstances have come into my life to show me exactly what it is like to be the receiver of that mistake. Or to show me how I appeared to others, or protect me from harm.

I personally have had an inordinate amount of experiences where people come into my life for a reason. I am not religious and do not believe it's God who is protecting me. During my lifetime, many interesting things have happened to me that give me the impression we do not have free will. Or, at the very least, there are things and circumstances that are bound to happen regardless of whether we have free will or not.

There are forces looking out for, or reprimanding, each individual human and humanity collectively. There are happenings and people in our lives for a reason. Without a doubt there is something more to this life than what it seems. That I know for certain.

I Have Seen The Future More Than Once, And I Am Not Alone

I'd like to share some personal examples that have time and again proven these ideas to me. I know I am not the only person who has had similar experiences. Often people will attribute these types of experiences and situations to "intervention" by God. This attribution to God I think is built more from simplicity of thought rather than truth. Questioning why and not having a concrete answer, that's difficult. It's easier for the mind to process by simply saying, "It was God's will."

The Plane Crash

In September 2007 I was heading to Bangkok, Thailand. Before I left I had a really weird anxious feeling. I told my friend, "I think I am gonna die in a plane crash on this trip. Either that, or it's going to be the best trip ever." Something weird was up.

At this point in my life I had flown from NYC to Japan and back more than ten times already. I'd been living in Tokyo and doing photo jobs in NYC since 2002. I had also been flying to Bangkok twice a year on average since that time. My flight status was a platinum mileage club member. I had flown over 100,000 miles since I turned twenty-one.

So flying and long haul flights never really bothered me. I would party all night, the night before and sleep the whole flight. Usually, I was sleeping before take off. This trip to Bangkok, however, when I boarded the plane my palms were all sweaty. I was anxious and I didn't sleep the entire flight.

During the descent and landing in Bangkok I was again very anxious and had sweaty palms. The landing ended up being routine and we arrived in Bangkok without issue. I breathed a sigh of relief.

My schedule had me staying in Bangkok for two days. With a final destination of Phuket. At the time I was doing a lot of travel photography and had made some friends in Phuket. So I would go for about one month each time. It was a good excuse to relax at the beach.

From Bangkok To Phuket

To get to Phuket from Bangkok you can either fly, which takes about ninety minutes, or take a twelve hour bus ride. Flights were cheap back then. Still feeling unsure about flying, I had placed a twenty-four hour hold on a ticket with a travel agency after my arrival.

I woke up the morning of my flight feeling really anxious about flying. I decided to be safe rather than sorry. I canceled my reservation and went to the bus station. I had done the bus ride before. It's really cheap and can be a bit harrowing.

The bus is a double decker and goes from evening overnight, for an early morning arrival. The air conditioning is on full blast, the drivers drive really fast, swerve often and break hard. It's not uncommon to wake up suddenly and think you are about to die. Not to mention the bathroom is super gross and the seats are cramped.

Still to this day when I recount this story it gives me chills. The bus finally pulled up to the loading area and everyone filed in. I stowed my bag in the overhead compartment, sat down in my seat and took a deep breath, sighing in relief. Bangkok is pretty hectic and I had been sitting in the hot, smelly, outdoor bus station for a couple of hours.

On these buses each seat has a little TV like on the airplane. I turned on the TV right after letting out that huge sigh. Breaking News! A plane has just crashed in Phuket. I am literally watching the live footage of the plane I had a reservation on, in flames on the runway! My jaw just dropped, I couldn't believe it.

Did I Cheat Death?

Suddenly, my phone starts blowing up and my friends in NYC are calling to check if I am alive. This type of thing is a surreal experience and you can't really place how you feel in this situation. Almost ninety people died. Are you getting a second chance? Did you cheat death? I still wonder sometimes. Do I have some purpose now?

I personally wasn't on the plane so I didn't experience the trauma first hand. There's a bit of cognitive disconnect. I was in disbelief, but at the same time was relieved and slept most of the bus ride. But I couldn't help feeling slightly guilty, like could I have saved people? I thought to myself, OK it happened, you knew before it happened something would, but how could you be sure it would happen? At least now it has come to pass.

After I get to Phuket. I settle in, take a nap, and have a swim. Still in disbelief, I went to this really relaxed beach bar I liked to hang out most nights. It is on the South end of Kata beach and built into this huge old tree that must be hundreds of years old. I am not sure if it is still there anymore, but that was the spot to go back then.

Synchronicity

While I was having my drink I started talking to a guy sitting next to me. We got to talking about the plane crash. Before I could tell him my story he told me that he was one of the few people that survived the crash!

What a crazy coincidence. Even more, I'm shocked at how nonchalant he is talking about it. He said since he was seated next to the emergency door, he was one of the first people off the plane. I'm thinking, this guy is even luckier than me! Six hours after the plane crashed he is sitting at a bar, next to me. Less than a week after I had a premonition that there would be a plane crash. What are the chances?

Turns out the chances are apparently quite good that people like us are drawn together. On a later trip to Koh Tao, in 2010—a small, beautiful island in the Gulf of Thailand which you can only get to by boat—I met a girl and we started telling each other some of our crazy life stories. She told me about how she had a plan to fly to Phuket but decided not to go at the last minute. And that the plane crashed. She couldn't believe how lucky she was to be alive.

I naturally was very surprised to hear this story and I asked her, "What year?" Turned out it was the same flight! When I told her my story we were both really questioning how the Universe works. The next day she invited me to her house and showed me her ticket. She said she had saved it as a reminder of how lucky she is to be alive.

We shared this common energy and somehow it had brought us together. This wasn't the only time I would see the future. I have a few more energetic examples that elicit how the Universe works in mysterious ways.

9/11 Changed My Life Trajectory

In 2001 I was living in the East Village of New York City. At the time I was working as a photographer and doing some modeling on the side. I'd also been working with model agencies doing test shoots for up and coming models.

In the late Summer of 2000, Boss models asked me to shoot a new girl. Her name was Omahyra Mota. I was the first photographer she ever worked with. I photographed her in her boyfriend's military fatigues in Greenpoint, Brooklyn.

In February 2001 German Vogue published a few of my photos of Omahyra. After those photos were published she became world famous.

Things were going really well and my career was taking off. Then 9/11 happened.

I witnessed it first hand. Not only did I watch the planes hit the towers, I also watched the towers collapse from my rooftop. At that point I grabbed my camera and ran down there to take photos.

I snuck past the police line and what a sight. I will never forget it. After experiencing that first hand. I thought maybe it was a good time for me to go live abroad. The first industry to get cut in an economic downturn is the Arts. After 9/11 more than half of my work dried up. So I decided to move to Tokyo, Japan. But first I would go to the beach and relax.

My First Trip To Thailand

In October 2001, on a whim I bought a ticket to Thailand. Living in NYC in the aftermath of 9/11, I need a break from the drumbeat of war. So during the second week of November I flew to Bangkok.

A few days after I arrived I was having drinks in the tourist area known as Khao San road. I had no idea where to go in Bangkok at the time. Back then Bangkok wasn't the developed cosmopolitan metropolis it is now. I had planned to stay only a few days in Bangkok to see the sights and head to Phuket for three weeks to sit on the beach and process what had just happened in America.

Late one night I chatted up this girl that was walking past me on Khao San road. She said, "I am headed to my friend's bar. If you want to talk to me, come along." So like a puppy I followed her. It was getting late, about one in the morning.

We sat and had one drink, talked for maybe thirty minutes and then, like a girl who is gonna turn into a pumpkin, she ran off to go home. I was in love. She was then and still is now, very beautiful. I remember saying out loud to myself, "This is the girl I want to marry."

All I knew was her first name: Tibb. She told me she was an actress. And that's how I entered her name in my phone, Tibb, Tibb-Actress. We texted for a day or two and then she stopped replying.

Ten Years Later

Flash forward to 2011. I am in NYC at a bar / music venue called Union Pool in Brooklyn. At the time I smoked cigarettes. My friends had just left and I was also about to leave. But first I wanted to smoke a cigarette.

I took a look outside in the smoking area and saw a cute girl with bangs and bob cut, sitting alone. I walked up and sat down next to her and asked her for a cigarette. She introduced herself as Tibb, told me she was from Thailand and had just moved to NYC. We hit it off right away. Something about her felt very close and familiar but I couldn't place it.

We ended up dating and spending a lot of time together. After a few weeks I realized it was her! The same girl I met ten years earlier in 2001 on Khao San road. Of course she didn't believe me, but said she did remember meeting an American guy on Khao San road one time, and she used to hang out there often when she was in university.

Back To Thailand

After five months of dating, Tibb's visa expired and she had to go back to Thailand. She invited me to come with her. On a whim I followed her. This is actually the story of how Pure Luck Bangkok was born. The two of us ended up opening Thailand's first ever kombucha brewery in Chinatown, Bangkok in 2013.

After living in Thailand for a few months, one day we were driving past Khao San road. So I asked her to take me to her friend's bar where she used to hang out. She said it was closed now but we could go anyway. She walked us through the very same alleyway we went through together in 2001. Directly to stop and stand in the exact spot under a tree where she sat the night we had our first drink together.

I said to her, "I was right!" She said with a laugh, "I remembered the guy's name was Jason." Then I said, "you told me you were an actress," and she confessed that she used to tell guys back then that she was an actress. "I knew it was you!" I laughed. "I can't believe it."

Right there, I told her how, that night, after she left, I wished that we would be married. She laughed at how it came out of my mouth. At the time neither of us believed in marriage. Somehow the Universe had brought us back together. Whether I willed it, or it was meant to be who can be sure. However, there's more to our story, which makes me lean toward the latter.

The Car Crash

In Thailand many families have their own personal Psychic. After a couple years of living together in Bangkok. One night we are having dinner and Tibb tells me that her mother had been to see their Psychic.

He told her mother that something tragic could happen to Tibb soon. He specifically said it could be a car crash and she might die. After breaking this unsettling news to me. She proceeded to run off all the times that this Psychic had predicted things for her family and they had come true.

Thailand is quite a mystical country and after living there for eight years and having traveled there for twenty I could definitely feel the air of mysticism. I got into the habit of burning incense at the temples and saying Sanskrit prayers and attended temple ceremonies New Years day with her family and so forth.

Tibb was the person who taught me to meditate. Her father wakes up at three in the morning every day to meditate and she had been meditating since childhood. You can see it in her aura. She is also the sweetest, kindest woman I have ever known. But she is Thai after all, so don't make her angry! I seem to have a knack for that.

One day in 2015, I was in NYC working and Tibb was in Bangkok. She is a designer and had been freelancing for a Thai-based fashion brand. The brand was having a launch party for a new collection Tibb created. 2 Many DJ's (the act) were headlining the event. It was set to be a rager.

The Russian Guys

Around 1 a.m. Bangkok time I received a call from Tibb. She was leaving the party and called me because she was in the parking garage and couldn't find her car. There were three Russian guys, who were also at the party. They were trying to get her to go in the car with them. I could hear them in the background and she showed me on FaceTime. I saw one girl with them who could barely stand up and looked like she was gonna fall over.

Tibb said these guys kept bringing her glasses of champagne. That she was dancing on the turn turntables, and that she wanted me to keep her company and safe. I asked her to face the phone towards the Russian guys. I told them to leave her alone and then she did the same.

We walked around the garage together and finally she found her car. This is the thing about Thailand, a single girl late at night is not safe in a taxi. Not to mention the Russian guys were still lingering. I could hear them in the background still calling for her to come with them.

The Drive Home

Tibb got in her car while I was still on FaceTime. Put her phone in the holder behind the steering wheel where the speedometer is. This is something we always did when she was driving. Because in Bangkok, you are always in the car. I obviously wanted to make sure she gets home safe and if something did happen I would be able to call her family right away.

Tibb has a very strong constitution and is quite strong willed. Plus, she is a master at driving in Bangkok. She learned how to drive in Bangkok. I was less concerned about her skills at that point and just wanted to make sure those guys didn't follow her home.

As she was driving she started acting really uncharacteristically strange. Crying then nodding off, eyes closed, like she was gonna pass out. So I am yelling as loud as I can, "WAKE UP! PAY ATTENTION!" and she would snap out of it, and then again it's the same thing. We go through the cycle about three times. Each time her eyes close like she is going to pass out. I have to yell as loud as I can to wake her up. Luckily, the house was only a ten minute drive and there wasn't any traffic or cars on the road.

After she arrives home and locks the door. In the middle of a sentence she drops the phone on the bed, falls on the bed herself, and passes out with me still on FaceTime. I was very concerned that the Russian guys spiked her drink, but there was nothing more I could do. I stayed on the line for about an hour and sent her a text to call me when she woke up.

The Investigation

The next day she didn't remember a thing. Not even speaking to me for almost an hour. She thought she may have been roofied. In case you are unfamiliar, roofies are called the date rape drug. Because they make you pass out and forget everything that happened.

I concurred and we agreed she should do some investigating. Bangkok is a really small place if you roll in certain circles. Everyone knows each other. They all went to the same international schools and all the "farang" or foreigners stand out like a sore thumb.

A few days later we found out that a girl at that party had been roofied and sexually assaulted. There were also multiple stories of girls claiming they had been roofied. We then found out that the guys trying to make

Tibb go in the car with her were small-time Russian mafia drug dealers. It turns out they were the ones spiking everyone's drinks.

Her Psychic was right. A tragic event could have happened but thanks to our energetic entanglement we were fortunate enough to steer past it. It's very unlikely she would have gone with the Russian guys. But had I not been on the phone it's very likely she would have passed out while driving and crashed her car. I feel very grateful for her in my life and still to this day am glad I was able to help her avoid harm.

Eighteen Years After We First Met

Tibb and I have been through a lot together. Eighteen years from when we first met my wish came true. We were married in 2020. I strongly believe that our paths crossed for a reason. We are meant to save each other's lives from tragedy. Had 9/11 never happened my life would have turned much differently!

Still to this day our influence on each other's lives is very strong. She too has saved my life. It was her that helped me stop being an alcoholic. This book wouldn't be possible and I wouldn't be here today if I didn't borrow that cigarette from her back in 2011. In 2001 our energies were entangled and some future strokes of fate were written.

My Dream About The Pandemic

In 2017 we were in Bangkok. Tibb was sitting on the bed next to me doing work on the computer. It was the middle of the day and very hot outside. Heat makes me lazy and so I nodded off to sleep. During this nap I had a prescient dream.

In my dream, it was a beautiful sunny day. Tibb and I were sitting on a big rock, while a beautiful clear river flowed by us on both sides. The sun glittered off the water and the whole scene was serene and peaceful. I woke up and told Tibb, "I just had the weirdest dream. We were sitting on a rock, in a river, in Ojai,… during a pandemic!" She responded, "What's a pandemic?" and blew me off as usual. "Whatever, you always have weird dreams" and she went back to work on her computer.

To this day I remember the image of us on the rock in this dream so clearly. I thought how strange it was in my dream. I not only knew there was a pandemic, but also that the rock we were sitting on was in Ojai.

For a minute, I kinda thought it was ominous but I didn't really think much of it. Not until 2020, when we moved to Ojai, California, and were sitting on the exact same rock in my dream during a pandemic! The whole dream experience came flashing back.

The day, the bed, and me telling Tibb and being really perplexed that I knew there was a pandemic. Turns out the river was the Ventura river which runs through Ojai. The Oso Hiking Trail where the river runs through the Ventura River Preserve is five minutes from our house and we go there all the time to lounge in the water, and pick sage and wild fennel. We had been to Ojai before I had my dream, but never to the spot in the river I dreamt about.

The Universe Sets The Direction, One Can Only Steer Ever So Slightly

Ojai is where I finally put pen to paper. For a long time I felt as though I should write this book. Which makes me wonder if this book was already written by the Universe in me. I can't help but think. Was this whole situation just a force to bring it to life?

Why did I have that dream? What did it foreshadow? There was no conclusion in the dream. And how could I know it was during a pandemic when it was just the two of us and a river? Who gave me the knowledge? Did I wake up too soon to get the entire message?

I feel like my life was reset in Ojai. In many ways Tibb and I both started over. We discovered ourselves so much deeper than we had ever before. I believe the pandemic forced many people to confront themselves. To rethink what it means to be honest with ourselves.

When a computer gets glitchy, the first advice any tech will give you is to turn it on and off. To reset it. If you pay attention to the verbiage being used by world leaders you will also see that the 2020, 50th annual meeting of the World Economic Forum was called "The Great Reset."

Resetting Ourselves

The first step in resetting anything is to wipe the slate clean. I do not mean to destroy the physical world that we have built. My meaning here is being honest with ourselves. We must look at ourselves, our life and our behaviors with a critical and objective eye.

In order to mentally rebuild a new world with our minds. By creating a new way of thinking from the inside out. Changing our thinking will change the world before lifting a finger. The best we can do is to control our thoughts and stay calm. Thoughts can and will become our worst enemy. Thoughts can create, or recreate, our futures.

The negative effects of thoughts on the body alone are enormous. There are countless studies that prove this. Depression actually shrinks the size of the human heart. We must be honest with ourselves, and also with others.

Society is built on trust. However, this foundation of trust has eroded and is continuing to erode very quickly. Trust must begin to be rebuilt inside ourselves. We must own our failures as much as our accomplishments.

The Network Of Our Mind

Humans are not all knowing beings. Oh wait. Yes, we are! We are connected to the quantum field. The quantum field, simply put, is the energy that is in us and all around us. It is the fabric of our reality. It controls everything. An all knowing Universal Intelligence. Just like a giant mainframe computer without any wires.

To learn more about accessing the data, interacting with this field and use cases. I recommend a book called Breaking the Habit of Being Yourself, by Dr. Joe Dispenza. He makes the linkage to the quantum field approachable, scientific, and elegant. If all humans could master the methods he teaches, we could make change on a global scale rather quickly.

Focusing Thought

There is a lot of scientific evidence showing the strength of focused energy. One mentioned in chapter 7, the HearthMath Institutes studies. Another is called the Global Consciousness Project, at Princeton University. "The project uses devices called random event generators (REG's) that usually produce a continuous sequence of completely unpredictable numbers which can be recorded in computer files. Experiments have shown that human consciousness can make the string of numbers slightly non-random when people hold intentions to do so, or when there is a special state of coherent group consciousness. The difference is very small, but statistical analysis demonstrates that this correlation of the REG behavior with something about consciousness is real. It is as if our wishes could change the 50/50 odds of a coin flip ever so slightly."

Proximity to the REG did not matter. There was no distance too far to diminish the effects. Imagine fans at a stadium cheering on their team. There are many experiments similar to this one. They all tap into quantum mechanics and the quantum field.

Don't Let The Physical Rule You

Dr. Dispenza's book came into my life right at the moment I needed it most. For several years before (and during) Covid, I had been completely focused on rebuilding my body. I had a crick in my neck and my posture was terrible. Stemming from many years of sitting in a chair, using a pen and tablet editing photos or and projects.

My shoulder had formed a forward leaning posture but only on my right side. My hip was out of alignment due to an old kickboxing injury. I also had scoliosis since I was a teenager. Using yoga, diet, inflammation reducing CBD, acupuncture, exercise, and focused mediation, with determination I was able to overcome these physical issues.

The Other Me

Before I go any further. I want the reader to know: I was not always the incredibly health conscious person I am now. I have already mentioned it on several occasions but would like to elaborate further.

My mother never gave me junk food as a child. In university though, I started to fall off the wagon. Right after I turned 21 I began drinking rum and cokes in my classes. That progressed rather quickly to gin and tonics and finally my drink of choice, vodka martinis.

When you are an artist there are so many eclectic people hanging around who are—to put it bluntly—getting into weird shit. I owned an art gallery for a few years. Owning a gallery meant I could get beer and liquor sponsors. So there was a never ending supply of free booze and people who were happy to drink it with me. With that came distractions, parties, and party favors.

Being An Alcoholic

Alcoholism runs in my family. I never drank until I was 21. But from 21 until about 34, I was a heavy social drinker. If you have lived in New York City or Tokyo, then you know that almost every social function revolves around alcohol.

Many times the drinks are free (at least in NYC). I consumed copious amounts of alcohol 6-7 days a week and it took a toll on my mind. That much alcohol also really messed with my sleep schedule and my health.

I was pretty much mentally bankrupt. One time in Tokyo, I ended up at the police station and they made me take a breathalyzer. I blew .53. For reference, you are drunk driving if you blow .08 in most American states. Technically speaking, I should have died from alcohol poisoning that day. Really, I should have been dead, a second time! Not to mention, I was often experiencing alcohol induced depression and paranoia.

Kombucha Changed My Perspective

Luckily, I was able to snap out of it. As strange as it may sound, it was kombucha that started to get me healthy. And it was my wife Tibb that pulled me up over the rim. The probiotics in kombucha changed the way I viewed my body, my food, and the world around me. Kombucha actually changed my perspective.

When I turned 34 I decided to get my health back and rebuild my mind and body. So I stopped drinking ten cocktails a night. At first I limited myself to weekends. This was difficult and it would be many more years before I stopped drinking alcohol altogether. But at least I was making progress.

I still love the idea of fermentation and the flavors of wine and champagne. These days I feel so good every day. I never have problems sleeping. I have lots of energy and my mind is as sharp as it's ever been. Just the thought of a hangover is enough of a deterrent to stop me from drinking.

During the time period when I was thinking now is the time to try to clean up my act, kombucha was this new thing. Just out in New York City from California. I was drinking it to cure my massive hangovers.

Tea, And By Extension Kombucha

As synchronicity would have it, my roommate in Brooklyn bought a kombucha kit to make kombucha at home. Inspired by her, I started making my own kombucha. Originally, what was for personal consumption grew into an art project born from my love for tea - tea being one of the most simple and energetic strings throughout history. Hence the first chapter in the book. Tea was also the first chapter in my sobriety.

I was feeling the mood lifting effects of kombucha. The connection it gave me to my body and the realizations mentioned above. This all made me think that if everyone in the world drank kombucha—not the sugary sweet kombucha like many brands today, but properly long fermented, without added sugars—Earth would be a better place. Properly made kombucha really does improve mood and energy levels. It makes humans happy and almost forces you to become aware of your diet and your body. This is all thanks to the gut brain connection.

From My First Batch To Top 5 In America

I made my first batch of kombucha in 2010. Three gallons of a single flavor, peach. Using white peony tea with a peach blend. I fermented this kombucha in an old brown, three gallon, glass milk jug that I found at a place called the Junk Store on Berry Ave. in Williamsburg, Brooklyn. The kombucha was delicious and so well received by everyone who drank it. I decided to make it a business.

On my second go, I made eleven flavors, fifty-five gallons worth, which I sold at the Escape From NY music festival in the Hamptons. We called ourselves the Kombucha Party at the time. Then I opened NYC's first kombucha bar in Williamsburg on Metropolitan Avenue and named it Pure Luck Tea Bar. We sold 35 organic teas and 12 flavors of kombucha. What a fun time!

This is the origin story of my kombucha brand called Pure Luck®. In 2017 Food & Wine Magazine named us "Top 5 Best" in America. Pure Luck® has also become known as the "pioneer" of kombucha in Asia.

In 2013, we opened Bangkok's first ever kombucha brewery. In 2017, we opened the first dedicated kombucha school, also in Bangkok. People would visit us from all over the world just to try Pure Luck and take our classes. We have provided inspiration to countless people. It was, and still is amazing.

Pure Luck® - Pure Kombucha

Pure Kombucha™, as we call it, is quite complicated to make. Always organic, brewed in 20 liter glass jars with spring water. Depending on the flavor, it takes 60-90 days to make each batch, from brew to sale.

We let each bottle carbonate naturally, like proper champagne. Pure Luck® - Pure Kombucha is the only room temperature, shelf stable kombucha in the world that has a shelf life minimum of two years. You could leave a bottle of Pure Luck at room temperature for years and it will age just like wine, with subtle and enjoyable flavors.

However, we failed the test of scaling up. We had trouble convincing potential investors to help us grow the brand. Easy, large volume and fast are what potential investors were interested in. They always said we should use massive stainless steel fermenters and force carbonate. Make a million bottles a month.

This is not possible to do while keeping the same quality. Out of love for what we do, we have kept it boutique. As of 2024 Pure Luck Bangkok is still producing kombucha. It will be our Bangkok location's 12 year anniversary in 2025.

Unfortunately, the beverage business is a very expensive game in America. Margins are thin and it is a lot of work and stress. COVID forced us to shut our San Francisco brewery in 2020. In the end, I think this was more of a blessing than curse. It freed me up to sit for two years and write this book. Putting to use all that I learned in advertising, health, and wellness over the last few decades.

Kombucha Brought Everything Full Circle

Operating a kombucha brand had me laser focused on my body and my health. Yet, I couldn't help to feel like I was missing something in my journey to upright myself again. I was literally banging my head against the wall feeling stuck.

Normally, I was pretty good at connecting with the universe and manifesting things. As I mentioned earlier in this chapter I have some sort of gift that connects. I always have, my mother says I get it from her.

But for the last few years I felt like I was spinning my wheels. Then I came across Breaking the Habit of Being Yourself. This book made me realize the reason I was running on the hamster wheel, as Dr. Dispenza puts it. Was because I had been laser focused on my body, but I had forgotten about my mind.

Of course I meditated every day for many years. But, I was always focusing on my body. The reason I wasn't getting anywhere didn't hit me until I read this book.

The Mind Controls Everything, And Anything Is Possible

I needed to give the reins of control back to my mind. Because I was letting my body control everything and living too much in the physical world. Always focusing my meditation on healing my body. It took many years and tears to heal. I suffered a lot of healing crises.

Turns out, when your hips are out of alignment so are your knees, ankles and shoulders—everything in your body is connected. I limped and learned a lot. I am a much stronger person mentally and physically now.

What does all this have to do with honesty and our thoughts? For one, I want to be honest with the reader. It is work and dedication to make change. I wasn't always positive, calm, and health conscious like I am now.

I want to be honest and let everyone know that I used to be an alcoholic, who smoked cigarettes and cannabis every day. That feels like another person, and it was someone else. I was not a good person when I was younger and had karmic debts due.

The other point I want to make here is that the mind is what controls our reality, our future, and our body. For many years I was so caught up in healing my body. I had actually forgotten to focus on creating my future with my mind. I have, Dr. Dispenza, to thank for reminding me.

I believe that in order to have a clear mind, humans need to clear the body of toxins. In the end, it is both. You can't have one without the other. While keeping in mind that the mind controls the body. In my case I had let my body and the physical world become my bias. The physical world ruled my life. Finally, I snapped out of it and things started changing and have really improved since that point.

Biases Mostly Affect Us Negatively

Biases inform us. Sometimes to our benefit, but more often than not to our detriment. We must always question ourselves—our behaviors, intentions, thoughts, and motivations. Always check the reactionary code. Most often we manipulate ourselves more than we do others. This is good when we use our mind to manifest our future in a positive way.

However, if we follow a philosophy of never being wrong and doubling down when we are actually wrong. If we make poor decisions because our thought process has been hijacked or manipulated. Or because of a lack of honest objectivity. If we act solely to be seen as "strong" or to sell it to ourselves that things are not our fault. If we act like we are the victim.

These behaviors will never help us be better at being honest with ourselves. Nor will they build a stronger, more connected, equal society, self, and world. Every one of us must take ownership for all our individual and collective failures, as well as our wins.

Humans learn by failing and analyzing where they failed. We learn by repeating and adjusting. This is the most basic concept of how we evolve. Try, fail or succeed, analyze, adapt, repeat. This is the formula and why I think this life is meant for us to do the same on a metaphysical scale.

There is another formula. You may even be doing this yourself and be unaware. It goes like this. Deny, obfuscate and make excuses, blame the other. State victimhood. No ownership required when you are infallible and it's everyone else's fault. When there is always some excuse to make you feel better about yourself. To look better in your or another's eyes.

Telling ourselves we personally are correct and always a victim allows us mentally to free ourselves from the responsibility of our actions and thoughts. This configures the code for continuation of negative behavior.

Humans must take ownership because our life is a creation of the human mind. We individually are 100% responsible for our lives, no one else is. Someone important in my life once told me, "this life is not a dress rehearsal." This stuck with me. I hope it will stick with you too.

Our thoughts, beliefs, and honesty matter. We must be transparent inside and out. We must reflect our true selves to inspire others. You have to take ownership for everything in your life. Because you are the one creating it.

CHAPTER FIFTEEN

Mycelium

There are millions of different fungi species worldwide. Many of these are called micro-fungi. Yeasts, molds, and slime molds. There are about 15,000 macro-fungi, which grow mushrooms, puffballs, truffles, and the like. These are the fruiting bodies of mycelium. We can learn from this species.

Fungi are perhaps one of the oldest and largest organisms on this planet with a billion plus years of experience. Adopting and evolving through cycles of climate changes and global extinctions. Fungi have survived, growing massive, underground, intelligent, interconnected mycelium webs. These webs are used to transmit information and store carbon. They are an underground, neurological net co-existing with partners on the surface. Seeking carbon, mycelium gives an offering.

Fungi Are Reciprocal

There is an interesting, self reinforcing cycle at work here. Mycelium makes the offering. The mushroom (and many other forms) releases spores. The spores attract insects, in turn attracting birds, which bring seed and fertilizer from which plants grow. In return, the mycelium network receives carbon from the roots of the plants and decaying materials to feed, propagate, and grow.

Recent research suggests that, through the root systems, plants and trees use mycelium to communicate, share information, and exchange carbon molecules for nutrients. Without these mycelial networks silently living underground, Earth and humans may perish. They are essential to life on this planet. The fungi family comprises a percentage of the physical mass of your body, as already mentioned.

Man Has Been Eating Mushrooms Probably Since The Dawn Of Man

This is where it gets interesting. Spore producing organisms have been known to hack the brains of their hosts. Mushrooms are consumed by 23 species, including monkeys and humans. It's not a huge stretch to suspect humankind has been consuming mushrooms for pretty much most of our existence. Some mushrooms will heal you, some will kill you. Some will make you hallucinate.

As natural born naturalists—that is, a species who lives off of nature and is knowledgeable of the natural world—prehistoric species would be able to recognize the berries, mushrooms, or whatever in the environment that will kill them, feed them, heal them, or make them hallucinate.

Psychedelic Mushrooms

Anyone who has taken a psychedelic mushroom trip will attest there is this great sense of well-being and connected effect that is a bit difficult to explain. You get a sense of joy and confidence in connectedness with nature and the Universe.

You just feel like everything is going to be OK. Much like how I personally feel after meditating. I imagine the same can be said for others as well. The side effects are also similar to regular meditative practice. There are many studies that have proven the benefits of psilocybin, the chemical component in mushrooms that makes you trip.

After a mushroom trip, people report long lasting, positive mental side effects. Like happiness, empathy and connectedness. Clinical studies show that psychedelic mushrooms cure depression and PTSD. The theory is a psychedelic mushroom trip helps the human brain create new neural connections. Pruning old neural connections, helping to overcome past trauma.

Right now, humans are at the cutting edge of using psychedelics to treat people with depression and PTSD. Some states in America like Washington and Colorado have decriminalized psychedelic mushrooms, or magic mushrooms as people like to call them.

I personally contributed to the measure in Colorado. Being one of 5,000 people who signed the petition to get the decriminalization measure on the ballot. I was so happy to see it passed! I love Colorado. Psychedelics work very well, speaking from my experience. A mushroom trip can help you break through mental blocks.

My Own Experience

When I was younger, I was stuck on an ex-girlfriend. We had a bit of a tumultuous relationship. After we broke up it made me depressed. One day some friends and I ate some psilocybe cubensis. This is one of the most common forms of mushroom that will make you hallucinate. They have gold caps and a grayish stem with a bluish tint. The blueish tint is one way to identify if a mushroom contains psilocybin.

After I woke up the next day, the depression from my breakup was gone. It was amazing. For months I had been so depressed. And then overnight I wasn't depressed anymore. It was like magic. Of course this must be why these types of mushrooms are called magic mushrooms.

Growing Neural Pathways Enabling New Ways Of Thinking

There are about 180 species of mushroom that contain psilocybin, of which roughly 95 contain enough for a psychedelic trip. Research shows that psilocybin and other compounds present in these mushrooms help to grow new neural pathways.

Imagine that, pun intended, the fruiting body of the underground neural pathway of plants and trees helps the human brain grow new neural pathways! Enabling new ways of thinking.

Prehistoric man must have encountered a lot of conundrums. There were certainly many problems to solve for them. It's possible to theorize that eating mushrooms contributed to problem solving abilities and perhaps even led to the invention of speech and language. This theory is attributed to the synesthesia brought on by hallucination. When you hallucinate you often experience synesthesia.

Synesthesia And Evolution

Synesthesia is an association of colors or sounds stemming from hearing, or seeing colors, sounds, or other physical things. If you are unfamiliar with the term, search it for a better understanding.

Imagine you are a prehistoric human. You are stuck on a problem. You eat some of these mushrooms which help to have a creative breakthrough. Putting it another way, these mushrooms help with thinking outside of the box, spurring creative thoughts, new neural pathway growth, and changes in the brain. Helping to overcome blocks, or problems.

Now, imagine this occurring over a very, very long period of time. With each generation helping humankind solve more and more complex problems. Growing more and more neural pathways. Building systems to survive. Through synesthesia inspiring language and other means of communication. It becomes a self reinforcing process.

Mushrooms are about sharing and healing. Mycelium shares the mushroom with the creatures living above ground. In the natural world most species barter their existence. Imagine a flower and a bee, or fruits and monkeys, or berries and birds. They all give and get. Magic mushrooms are sharing with humans the intelligence and love of nature. But what are humans sharing back?

Mycelium Has Been Helping Plants Flourish For A Long Time

Fossil records suggest mycelium-like organisms have existed on this planet long before plants, possibly going as far back as 2.4 billion years. For all we know, mycelium could be some sort of intelligent alien race that colonized Earth way before humans arrived.

Scientists theorize, at some point in time above ground flora and the mycelium negotiated a mutually beneficial contract to work in synchronicity with each other to self-regulate and harmonize. Underground mycelium systems allow plants to flourish on Earth.

More plants growing above the surface creates more carbon and decay for the mycelial walls to grow below. Mycelial structures act like an internet to help roots of plants and trees share information and nutrients.

The plants above regulate the climate of the planet. It's possible to think of mycelium as the nerve system of the planet, recording and reading real time data about the climate and carbon make up of the atmosphere then redistributing it below. There is still much to discover here.

Broken Connections

For a long time modern humans have been told taking hallucinogens is bad. Leaving us collectively stuck mentally, and environmentally broke. To say we have lost the love and connection to the natural world is probably an understatement. Our upside-down approach has definitely made humanity lose this connection to the natural world. A connection ultimately required for our survival.

The Fungi Kingdom consists of organisms that break down matter from wood to animals to petroleum. Fungi has the power to transform dead decay into life. Mycelium is about giving and receiving. About rebirth and life.

It is not solely about taking, as humans are doing. Taking from the Earth humans give nothing in return. This way is out of balance. Nature will show us the way. We must simply observe and follow nature's lead.

CHAPTER SIXTEEN

Sick Care

Sick care is something that cannot be overlooked. In America, 70% of the population is considered overweight of which 30% is considered morbidly obese. Have you been to a hospital or doctor's office? If you have then you know they are selling fast food in the hospital. I don't think I need to discuss how harmful fast food is.

What about jello? Hospitals serve jello to inpatients. What you may not be aware of is that jello contains numerous food dyes and artificial sweeteners with known carcinogenic effects. Once again, this is the upside-down world. What about getting a lolly pop at the dentist? One time a dentist joked to me, "It's job security." This comment is the upside-down world at its most honest.

The Healthcare Industry Itself Is Not Healthy

Would you consider the Healthcare Industry workers or the industry itself to be healthy? The paperwork alone is enough to drive you mad. I do not write this to bash anyone, just to make a point. Many, if not most in this industry work grueling, long shifts and are unable to maintain proper sleep cycles. The opportunity to have a regular, balanced rhythm, and eat properly, on a normal schedule, must be almost non-existent. Not to mention the high stress levels.

When I go to the doctor, if almost everyone that works in the office is overweight and does not look healthy. And the food served at hospitals is known to have negative effects on the human body. When, often people who work in health care are not able to have a healthy lifestyle themselves. When there are fast food chains in the hospital—I'm not sure how we can call this health care. If the patients are sick and the staff are also not healthy, shouldn't we be calling this sick care?

Health Care Reflects Our Collective Well-being

This is not only limited to the "health care" industry. This is the majority of peoples' jobs and lives. Look to health care for an example of our collective well-being. Imagine it from a marketing perspective. When you think of a doctor, what's the first mental image that you imagine a doctor looks like? Do you imagine a healthy, authoritative person? When you see advertisements for doctors and hospitals, they usually feature authoritative types.

Yet, when you get to the hospital or the doctor's office, many of the doctors and staff do not appear authoritative to me. Taking the time to put my well-being and health first, before money or anything else. I feel I must be an outlier.

Looking at it another way. If I'm buying a health drink, and the person selling it to me doesn't look healthy, I'm concerned. I feel the same way at the doctor's office.

If The Doctor Is Unhealthy It's Hard To Believe In The System

There isn't really any way to make this blunt statement sound better. When I go to the doctor and the doctor is obese or really doesn't look healthy. I look around the hospital and 70% of the employees are overweight, I can't help but feel concerned.

I know that these people don't have the opportunity to live a balanced life. It is also concerning seeing drugs advertised on TV with a long list of possible, insane side effects. I can't help but to think this is not a healthy system administering health.

From the top to the bottom. Policy to administration, everything is upside-down. Medicines have literally been engineered to make you sick. Just read the side effects. What more is there to say?

Millions Blindly Trust This System

The FDA says it's OK. Millions of people will take prescription drugs and give them to their children and pets! In 2021, as mentioned previously, 55% of the US population took prescription meds every day. One reason pharmaceuticals are pervasive in our water supply is because so many people are taking them daily.

Trusting unhealthy people to administer health doesn't sit right with me. How many of the doctors and health care workers take these very pills? How many get paid perks to administer them? If one of the side effects is sudden death, could this even be considered the administration of health?

Trusting Unhealthy People To Make Healthy Decisions

How can we count on unhealthy people to make healthy decisions? Look at how much sick care costs in America. The prices are outrageous. So very many decisions are made with only profits in mind.

Think about it. If humans keep humans sick, it's job security. Sick care is an incredibly massive industry. There will be more profits by keeping people sick. The insurance companies and the healthcare industry have inordinate amounts of money to lobby politicians.

True Story

A while back a colleague told me a story about their parent who is a heart surgeon. I've known this family for a long time. At the time this surgeon was recognized as one of the top in their field with many awards. This surgeon's services were in great demand, having an exemplary record of completing surgeries without complications or follow up visits.

This colleague told me how their parent was called into the hospital directors office and told to stop being such a good surgeon. The hospital wanted more complications and follow up visits. The surgeon, being a good person, was rightly upset and refused.

It was truly disconcerting to hear this. However, I wasn't surprised. The world we inhabit is an upside-down world that places profits at the top and people at the bottom. When money is the only motivation for a business, you cannot trust that the right things will be done. You and only you must be responsible for your health and well-being.

CHAPTER SEVENTEEN

Consent

You might want to say this part out loud: I do not consent. I do not consent to being a machine of the corporation, the economy, politicians, or anyone or anything that wishes to manipulate me. Whether subtly or otherwise, against my free will.

You Are Not A Machine

I am not a machine and am only human. My physiology and psychology are not built to be a machine. I am not built psychologically to work like a machine, day in and day out. I do not consent to such constant bombardment of stress.

I do not consent to chemical and pharmaceutical contaminated foods and water. Nor do I not consent to living in a society that puts profits first and people last. I do consent to live in a society that only benefits the few at the expense of the many. I do not consent to the collection and sale of every micro-point of my data. Nor do I consent to being advertised to every minute I am awake.

I am not my job and can be whatever I choose to be. I choose kindness, compassion, and love over division, retaliation, and hate. My job does not own me, nor does it define who I am. I own my work. I will put my health, the environment and sanity before convenience and money.

I realize this may seem like an impossible task. Thing is, it won't happen overnight. But with inspiration and a concerted effort on your part. You could make your life much closer to this reality than you think. The key is to put your mind to it. And not giving up.

Take Your Self Back

The proverbial "they" will push your limits, milk you for every drop, and leave you hung out to dry. Take your self back. This is a fundamental change in thought that must take place. Throughout society, I think the COVID pandemic has helped in moving this shift of thinking back into the collective mindset.

Many people do not wish to go back to the old way, their old jobs, or back to the office. A record number of people have left the workforce and started their own business since COVID. Some may find out, as I did, this too can be incredibly stressful. Maybe even more so.

Many are searching for something more meaningful to do in their lives. To spend more time with their family or chasing their dreams. Realizing that life is fleeting. I would never have had the time to write this book if it were not for COVID.

I Want To Be Free To Express My Self

When you are a child the question is always, what do you want to be when you grow up? The answer should be I want to be creative, innovative, and free to express my self in a way that is fulfilling, engaging and interesting to me.

We must take back our self worth. When meeting someone, we address ourselves as what we are, not who we are. More often than not, the first question everyone asks is, "What do you do?" We live in a culture of classism and judgment through work titles. Not only how we define ourselves through our work, but how others make a first impression in their mind of you as well.

Nowhere is this more prevalent than in NYC (and LA). As a professional photographer I experienced this firsthand. Everyone immediately assumed I was the stereotype of my profession. Before being able to speak a second sentence they would always say, "So you only date models right?" I must have heard it thousands of times.

You Are Not Your Job, Give Yourself More Credit

In our current social setting, we meet and say, hi, my name is... I am a lawyer. I am a secretary. I am a plumber. Why do we give ourselves so little credit? We are not our job. Our sole reason to exist in this life is not just to be a machine to work for a corporation, or anyone besides your self. We are here to work on ourselves and our personal energetic needs. To contribute to a greater well-being, to learn, grow, and evolve.

If you truthfully love your job and are happy doing it and feel great about it, then you are working for your self. Maybe this is your purpose. Overall, I believe, most peoples' greater purpose has been hijacked.

When I lived in Tokyo I found it refreshing that when meeting people they would often ask, or talk about, their hobbies as part of a conversation starter. In a culture of such strong conformity and commitment to work. I saw this as a way for people to be seen as individuals.

Consent Should Be Mandatory

Do you believe in free thought? Free will? The right to eat chemical free food? Breath clean air? How about consent? I do not consent to being manipulated by corporations, politicians, advertisements, bacteria, pharmaceuticals, or chemicals.

I do not consent to eating chemically laced foods. I do not consent to live in a society that is being manipulated at the expenses of the energetic work and actual worth of each individual human. At the expense of the greater good. The expense of our own personal evolution.

Basic Human Rights

We live in a richly developed society now. We have the technology, know-how, and financial means to make certain that every human has shelter, water, safety, and clean food. These should be basic human rights. Why would anyone argue against this?

A human who has an opinion that one human is better than the other, from a purely monetary perspective, and does not deserve these basic necessities should be ashamed. What type of human is so selfish and willing to tread all over another as to deny anyone these basics?

Being Homeless In NYC

I personally had a very rough patch with alcoholism and had been homeless in New York City in winter. It was really just terrible timing. One week before the great recession of 2008, I spent my entire savings on new photo equipment and much needed dental work. Then the crash happened and I lost my job within the same two week period.

I experienced the psychological toll of lacking necessities firsthand. I had $30,000 worth of camera gear. Yet, I found myself homeless in my thirties, unable to meet the most basic necessities. It was just an unfortunate hand I was dealt at that time.

With no family to call on and everyone else in panic from the crash. I was forced into being homeless at night and sleeping on friends' couches during the day, while they were at work. The psychological toll is not easy to overcome. Still to this day I can feel the survival mindset.

Existing In A Scarcity Mindset

When COVID hit, we were forced to shut down the San Francisco brewery because our partners went bankrupt. The feelings and PTSD of not having regular income again were all too familiar. Humans who are not wealthy are not the lazy freeloaders many politicians portray them to be. They are just like everyone else. With the exception of a mental scarring from lost dignity and safety. No one should suffer homelessness in America. We are the richest country in the world.

Our most basic, yet weighted, stress comes from the worry of maintaining a roof over our head and having food to eat. Food, shelter, water, safety, and sanitation. In this modern society, it should be everyone's right.

If we do not stand up now. We may lose all control of free will, and eventually free thought. Already we see how those in power are trying to repress free thought through threats, book banning, bullying and coercion, erasure and surveillance. Right here in America. The future could be scary, but it doesn't have to be.

Living Environment Token

One possible mechanism could be to create a Living Environment token in lieu of fiat money. This would be a government backed, tokenized blockchain based crypto currency. Used exclusively to pay rent, make purchases at thrift shops and second hand shops and to pay for groceries.

It's not Socialism. It is a Living Environment and recycling in one. It would also spawn new businesses, economies, and opportunities. It would uplift millions of people, freeing their minds to feel like they are also part of society.

There is already a system for food and housing. Simplify it, demystify it, and reduce the bureaucratic burden and waste. We could be creating programs for landlords, grocers, and second hand shops to redeem blockchain based tokens for fiat money. This program could be open to all persons with income below a certain threshold—of x dollars per year net. Those above this level will not be eligible and for those below, opting in would be a choice.

Tax Free Income

As an incentive to landlords and businesses, these purchases could be entirely tax free income to accept. It would be direct, transparent, easily redeemable, and backed by the government. If you have traded cryptocurrency, then you know how easily achievable this is. Using a simple system connected to a bank account and converting LE, Living Environment tokens into USD.

Each token receiver and recipient would have a registered wallet identifier. Since every transaction is traceable and public (not by name, but by alphanumeric ID) on the blockchain. This would be efficient and eliminate fraud. Instead of outsourcing to a private company the government could be the sole source of conversion from LE to USD. It is not rocket science. It is caring, kindness, and equality.

The Benefits Will Be Huge

Having an LE token to pay for the basic needs of citizens would bring petty crime down and also reduce government waste. It would lift many from poverty and lower the collective stress levels of hundreds of millions of people.

Implemented in conjunction with better regulations regarding food, chemicals, and water quality. The citizenry would be well on its way toward being happier and living a longer, better quality of life. Society as a whole would benefit greatly.

Do not let anyone tell you this idea is radical or call it Socialism. It is neither. It is a guaranteed Living Environment. Thanks to the psychological impact on people and communities, a LE token would lead to new inventions, more wealth creation, a happier populace, higher employment, a higher birth rate, longer lives, and a stronger economy. It will also help in reducing waste through recycling second hand merchandise more efficiently. I strongly feel there is currency in caring for people. Anyone who fights against this is just a hater.

CHAPTER EIGHTEEN

Human Adaptability

We are born into this paradigm; it is all we know. The most amazing trait of the human condition is our malleability. Looking back throughout history on the plethora of different conditions and hierarchical structures humanity has been subjected to. One may conclude that any paradigm is possible.

Possible, that is, as long as the basic needs are met to sustain life. Food, water, safety, sanitation, and shelter. Being grand or not, if we are born into it, then it's all we will ever know. If everyone else is doing it, then we will do it too.

Setting The Paradigm

Governments, dictators, and corporations are aware of this. When you read a news article talking about the whittling down or erosion of, say, civil rights, or human rights. That translates into a long term strategic plan. In this plan, the infamous "They" know that tactically, over time, if they keep "eroding" what is universally understood as the current paradigm. Then those born into the new paradigm will not have known the old way and it will therefore be normal to them.

The Afghanistan Example

Take Afghanistan, for example. Now that the Americans have departed, the Taliban have seized back control of the country. Yet, there is one thing that has been problematic for the Taliban—twenty years of American rule. Under this rule, the minds and behaviors of an entire generation of Afghans born in the 1990s, or come of age during that twenty-year period have been changed.

Many in the media are calling this war a failure. Which it was. But there are always silver linings. An entire generation and more of the population, many of which are now into adulthood, have known only one paradigm. The American one. Where freedom and freedom of thought were allowed.

Women and girls could be educated and work, take part in the government, and live on somewhat more equal terms with men. Already there have been protests and people are fighting back.

To know freedom and have it taken away is much more powerful than to never have known freedom at all. That's the catch and that's human psychology—fighting harder to keep something than to gain it. This is a crack in the veneer of the new paradigm the Taliban wish to impose.

Chaos Creates Opportunity For The Power Hungry

It's a timely example of exactly what we see going on the world over. Authoritarian takeovers and major crackdowns on civil liberties, human rights, and basic freedoms of movement and thought. Many authoritarian leaders lately have taken the pandemic as their cue to crack down further and increase their powers of control.

In late 2021, it became known that one of the most prominent actresses in China had literally been erased from all searches, online mentions, and movie titles. She is at once famous, and yet now she does not exist. China has done this to its political prisoners as well. No record of them ever being arrested or taken to trial exists. They have simply disappeared.

For what crime? Speaking their own thoughts. Not thoughts that China wishes for its citizens to have. The current regime in China has a mighty, micro-managing approach to how its people should exist and think. Many fear this is only just the beginning of a New World Order.

The Malleable Mind And Body

Malleability applies not only to the world we live in and the rules that govern us. It also can be applicable to our personal perceptions of reality and our physical bodies in a myriad of ways. One important possibility is the ability to control your body and thoughts with your mind, breathing and meditation. Many real world examples of this exist.

Known as the "Ice Man" for his ability to withstand freezing cold temperatures. Take Wim Hof as an example. He teaches the Wim Hof Method. In essence his method is a series of breathing exercises. Using this method combined with meditation he is "able to voluntarily influence his autonomic nervous system." To suppress immune response.

I personally have used the Wim Hof method and it works. In my case I was able to withstand cold water temperatures much longer than I had ever been able to before. But like everything, this takes practice. The most important thing we can learn is how to control our mind.

Another example can be found in deep water divers who control their heart rate. This skill enables them to dive deeper than the average person. Holding their breath for very long periods of time through the sheer act of will power, practice, breath work, and focus.

Like any muscle, your body and mind can be shaped and controlled. Through meditative practice, deep focus, study, critical thought, the elimination of chemical and bacterial hackers, and through physical practice. We can heal the heart, lungs, spine, brain, and more. We can even manifest things we want in the future solely by using quantum mechanics and the rule of collapsing the wave function.

Be Like Water

Being malleable inspires great flexibility. We can use this to our advantage if we allow ourselves to free our minds from the physical rigidity of what we perceive to be our only thought paradigm. Bruce Lee famously said he learned to "be like water" and "move like water." You too can, "think like water."

Scientific experiments have shown that, when trapped, water at the atomic level will actually change the physical bonding structures of its Hydrogen and Oxygen molecules. In essence, water is shape-shifting to escape containment.

At eye level we are able to observe water's fluid dynamics. Water is always changing with its containment and gravity, going with the flow. Water is a symbol for flexibility. Being like water mentally takes practice. Once achieved, it is very gratifying to live and be like water.

Don't Be A Stone

Unfortunately, many humans become trapped in rigid ways of thinking. They are living more like stones. Unable to expand thought horizons and unable to accept that others may have and want broader horizons. These stones want everyone else to be stones like them, imposing their own personal self limitations on others.

Why should others have freedom of thought and flexibility of mind when they won't? This message drones on from only those with selfish interest in mind. Do not think for yourself, be like we say you should be, do what we tell you to do, and that is all. Follow the book, the culture, the rules, and carry on the way it always has been. Do not rock the boat.

Those in power, those with only control on the agenda will be happy this way. The people will never be. There is a saying that goes something like, the tree that bends in the wind will weather the storm. Meaning that standing too upright against the winds of change could mean the tree will be torn from its roots.

Not going with the flow and being the rock that blocks the river only forces the water to erode and find alternate pathways around it. The rock and broken tree will be left behind. The wind and water progress forward as they wish.

An Open Mind Takes Practice

Creating a more flexible mind is something that comes with practice, patience, focus, learning and tolerance. To fully achieve this, a clear head and body free of toxins and addiction is necessary.

Once achieved, a flexible human mind is the most powerful tool available to us in history. A flexible mind has the ability and great benefit of being able to serve us and society. And not only society, but our personal mental well-being and our physical well-being.

When we control our mind, bodies, inputs, and our thoughts, and accept the reality that 99.99999% of everything around us is energy. Then we allow our mind to tap into the collective subconscious, into the quantum field of energy around us. We live in the flow of life.

Change The World

If we spend every day clean minded, meditating first thing in the morning or right before bed with intention. Focused on creating a positive mental image of the reality we want to live in. And millions of people are doing this regularly. The chances of manifesting the wavelength and bringing these ideas into reality are quite good.

If we all are simultaneously projecting into the future a collective, positive well-being. A heart centered idea of what we want the world to be. If we are all manifesting this new society, where caring and the environment have value. Where love, equality and kindness are the focus. Where human creativity and expression is a feature, not a bug. Then we will be able to flip the upside-down world back right-side up.

It is as simple as a collective change in our ways of thinking. Freeing up time from our busy schedules for the benefit of ourselves and our fellow humans. Focusing less on earning money and the ego, and more on earning positive merit. Putting your health first and paying positivity forward.

This way we will be able to rebuild ourselves from our most natural states, free of corruption, addiction, and toxic thinking. This moment in history is an inflection point. We must cast off the anchors and sail ahead into uncharted waters and create the waves of a new paradigm. Together we will leave the old one in our wake.

CHAPTER NINETEEN

Be Brave

Our environment is what shapes us. You probably noticed there are always fast food restaurants in low income areas, and markets like Whole Foods in wealthier neighborhoods. Once again, this is the upside-down world at its finest. A design meant to keep people under the thumb.

Availability Of Quality Food Sources

Studies conducted in low income neighborhoods have shown. Simply by having access to affordable, geographically near, healthy food sources people eat healthier. By creating access to farmers markets, or simply placing a vegetable stand locally, the residents of these neighborhoods chose to eat healthier. This change happened solely by creating more opportunities for healthy eating.

When there are more opportunities for healthy food and less opportunities for unhealthy food a shift occurs. This is so basic. If the food being offered to us in supermarkets is changed to be more healthy. Humans will eat healthier.

Diet is a strong factor in human behaviors such as aggression, anger and mental stability. Something as simple as healthy eating is able to bring about positive change in human personality traits.

Time To Make Change

Welcome to the Anthropocene. It's time to change the way we live, work, eat, and think. I sincerely hope that I have inspired you to look at your daily life and the world around you in a different and profound way. The collection of information in this book comes from my deep interest in learning, culminating more than two decades of knowledge I have collected in my "need for cognition."

I am also an idealist. However, let's be realistic. There is a lot of information to absorb. I am not expecting readers to just flip a switch and implement all of the above ideas and concepts into daily life in one go. With each day, if you make a concerted effort, over time it will add up. It takes many raindrops to fill a bucket.

It Took Me Years

I spent more than a decade researching and learning with focused determination to get where I am today. The last 4 years of which I spent enormous effort on small concerted, focused steps. In order to get my diet, systems and mind to an easy, manageable state.

Once you possess the knowledge, form the habit and create the neurological pathways. Traversing the path becomes a part of your being. Technique transcends consciousness. By reading this book, you have started with a bucket that is half full. With focus, will power, and dedication, you can achieve anything. The initial push takes the most effort. Once you make those first steps you will gain momentum. Once you have the momentum, the key is to keep the ball rolling.

Meditation Is Your Best Friend

First and foremost, if you want to get a better perspective, I strongly recommend daily meditation. If you have children, teach your children to meditate as well. Create a lifelong habit that will provide your kids enormous benefits as they grow older.

Set aside at least 30 minutes a day—an hour will be even more beneficial. Schedule your day around this part of your routine. Everyday, first thing when you wake up, or just before you go to bed. Carve out some quiet time and mindfulness for yourself and do this together with your kids, if you have children. You can do it!

There are so many benefits when you make meditation a habit. Once you meditate regularly and see the results you won't want to stop. There will be days when you will have to force yourself. Even after many years, there are still days when I have to force myself. But I am always grateful when I finish meditating. Those are the days meditating probably benefits me the most. After about a year it will be like riding a bike.

True Achievement Takes Purposeful Focus

Personally, I made a pact with myself. For 365 days I said I would meditate every single day. No matter how miserable or whatever I felt. In the end I missed only 2 days. Once, I was majorly hungover and the other was also because of drinking too much.

These days, I almost never feel that way when I wake up, and I haven't missed a day in years. Even if it's just 5-10 minutes of focused breathing with your eyes closed, on the train or anywhere. It's worth it. Meditating has become a part of my life. I couldn't take on my day without it.

On most days I meditate about 30 minutes every morning. Right after I wake up. I schedule my entire life around this habit. Of course things come up and sometimes I have to take the chance when I get it at any point in the day. However, for the most part I make changes built around owning my time for peace of mind in the morning.

Brief Background On Meditation

The act of mediating is about 2,600 years old, give or take. No one is sure. There are two distinct forms of mediation and processes. Western or Christian meditation and Eastern or Asiatic meditation. Western mediation is focused on reciting prayer and connecting with God. It's structured around the belief that there is one top down ruler. This is why many Christians associate meditation as a religion. In this form there are no specific body poses. The whole idea is centered around connecting with God.

On the other end of the spectrum is Asiatic or Eastern mediation. This form focuses on technique and emptying one's mind. When I speak of meditation, I am referring specifically to the Eastern or Asiatic style.

In the Asiatic tradition, posture is very important. The focus is on Enlightenment and Self-Realization, bringing clarity of mind, clearing away stress and distraction, focusing on breathing, becoming one with the energy in and around us, seeking out one's true self.

This style of mediation frees the mind, connecting the body and mind as one. In my case when meditating, old memories often pop up. I tend to liken this to cleaning out the storage unit of the mind. Usually, new ideas will pop into my head as well, or creative solutions will reveal themselves to problems I may have. Mediating has given me a much deeper sense of empathy that I did not possess previously.

Some Recommendations

If you are already meditating daily, I suggest picking up a copy of Breaking The Habit Of Being Yourself by Dr. Dispenza. Using his techniques will help you to further break down any limiting actions and thoughts and help to gain even more perspective.

The next step I recommend is to start detoxing. Cut out processed foods and pharmaceuticals. Learn more about your current diet. Read the ingredients and if you don't know what something is take the time and learn. Do the research.

The more you learn the better position you will be in. Significantly reduce your sugar and alcohol consumption, including processed sugars. Remember just because the box says sugar free, that does not mean it is sweetener free. It will be hard at first. Both sugar and alcohol are very addictive.

This is when willpower is your best friend. Don't give into peer pressure. Your true friends will support you. Anyone who tries to tempt you astray is doing so for their own benefit. Don't give them that pleasure.

While you are doing these above steps. You may want to see how you feel after detoxing from social media, TV, and the news. Pick two or three consecutive days in a week and simply don't log on. Turn off all notifications, including those pesky email ones.

You might find yourself feeling freer and happier than you have in a long time. Put the phone and tablet down. Use this "you" time to connect with nature, work on a project, or get into something focused, read a real book. I'm not talking about a trashy romance novel either. Read something that will inspire, educate, and feed your brain.

Some recommendations of books I like: Siddhartha, by Herman Hesse. You may have read Siddhartha in high school. Reading it again as an adult is much different. I've personally read it many times. It's a great book to accompany you on the journey you are about to undertake.

A few more; The Art of Happiness, by the Dali Lama, The Tipping Point or Outliers, by Malcolm Gladwell (I recommend any of his books, I have read them all), A History of the World in 6 Glasses, by Tom Standage, Guns, Germs and Steel, by Jared Diamond. Just to name a few. The idea is to read something that gives you perspective. There are many great books out there.

Being Kind And Good Makes You Feel Good

In your day to day life, smile at people and do good unexpected things without reason for reward. Help an old lady cross the street, so to say. You will find that by doing good, you will feel good. Try not to get bogged down in the stress of your day to day.

Remember the physical world is entirely energy. Don't waste your energy taking out your problems on the cashier who is already most likely having a bad day of their own. Or that driver who just cut you off.

Remember that every single human has their own stress and problems to deal with. When committing small acts of kindness you are stimulating joy inside yourself. Not only that, you are inspiring others to do the same. Lead by example.

I also recommend finding a close friend, colleague, or peer to take on these challenges together. It's always better to have someone on your team. You can support each other during times of weakness.

Some Hurdles To Consider

A few more things worth mentioning. If you are a weed smoker, regardless of what people say, smoking cannabis before meditation is not a good idea. You will never find a monk or the Dali Lama smoking a joint before they meditate and you shouldn't either.

Cannabis clouds your mind and affects your brainwaves. I would know. As a lifetime daily pot smoker. I actually quit smoking pot specifically so I would have better sessions mediating. And It worked immensely. You too will find significantly better results when you are clearheaded.

Something else to think about. In my case, the moon cycles affect my will power. They also seem to reflect up and down periods. This may not be true for everyone. But you probably have a cycle of your own. The moon does have some effect on humans.

In some circles, the new moon represents the time when it is darkest. This means that darker forces have more pull. Usually, in my case, if something bad is happening to me, for whatever reason it's almost always around the new moon.

Others view the new moon as a time of new beginnings. Just remember the new moon and the full moon are the most powerful periods to mediate and manifest. I make it a point to make extra effort and time to really drive home what my intentions are during these days of the month.

I downloaded an app on my phone. This helps me track the moon's cycle. When I start feeling less willpower, I check the app and the majority of the time it is close to the new moon. This helps me be able to tell myself that my lack of willpower is simply part of the cycle and to just get through the next few days.

This simple trick has been very useful for me. Everything is a cycle in this life. Becoming aware of the cycles and how you are personally affected will greatly help you succeed. I hope this book will give you tools to succeed and live a healthier life.

Learning Never Ends

If it were up to me, the things I write about here would be taught in every K-12 school possible. Learning is, and always has been, an integral part of succeeding at this life. Formal education gives only the bare minimum in preparation to live within the paradigm set for us. To continue the status quo, but not to live or think outside of it.

In this current iteration of the world. It is up to each individual to seek out the information that is being hidden from them. To not only discover information, but also to discover themselves. True self discovery is nuanced and unbiased. It does not just happen.

Each human has to make a conscious effort to discover their greatness and weaknesses. Just like any computer is a blank slate, so is the human brain at birth. Choosing the right programs, software, and hardware, uploading the right data and doing proper maintenance—these steps are all essential.

Treat your mind (and your gut) like you would your most precious assets because they are, after all, your most precious assets. Without them you are nothing but a shell.

Printed in Great Britain
by Amazon